CENTERING WITH MANDALAS: VOLUME 2

OVER 125 ADULT COLORING DESIGNS

BY
MARY ROBBINS

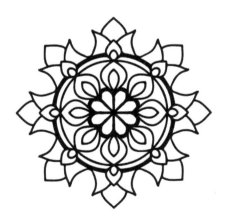

MENDED EARTH STUDIO

Centering is often used to describe a relaxed but focused state of mind. This process clears your mind of thoughts and worries about the past and future and brings your thoughts to the present moment. Taking time to add color to each of the mandalas in this coloring book will assist you in finding the center of your being. Your center is where natural creative and positive energy flows through you, instantly reducing anxiety and stress.

There is a tag included at the top of each of the 64 mandala coloring pages. You can use these tags in several ways: to write your name and the date, to track your completion of each page, to practice your coloring materials, and color choices before starting on a mandala. You can also color and cut them out to use as a gift tag, label, or bookmark!

We would love to hear from you! Visit our website to contact us with questions, comments, suggestions, or to share images of your completed coloring pages for a chance to be featured! You can find us on social media under the name: PatternsByMES. PatternsByMES is the branch of Mended Earth Studio that focuses on the digital design of patterns and graphics.

Designs and cover layout by Mary Robbins
Cover artwork colored by Mandy Blaney
Copyright © 2021 by Mary Robbins and Mandy Blaney
Copyright © 2021 by Mended Earth Studio
www.mendedearthstudio.com
All rights reserved.

International Standard Book Number
ISBN-13: 978-0-578-83218-0

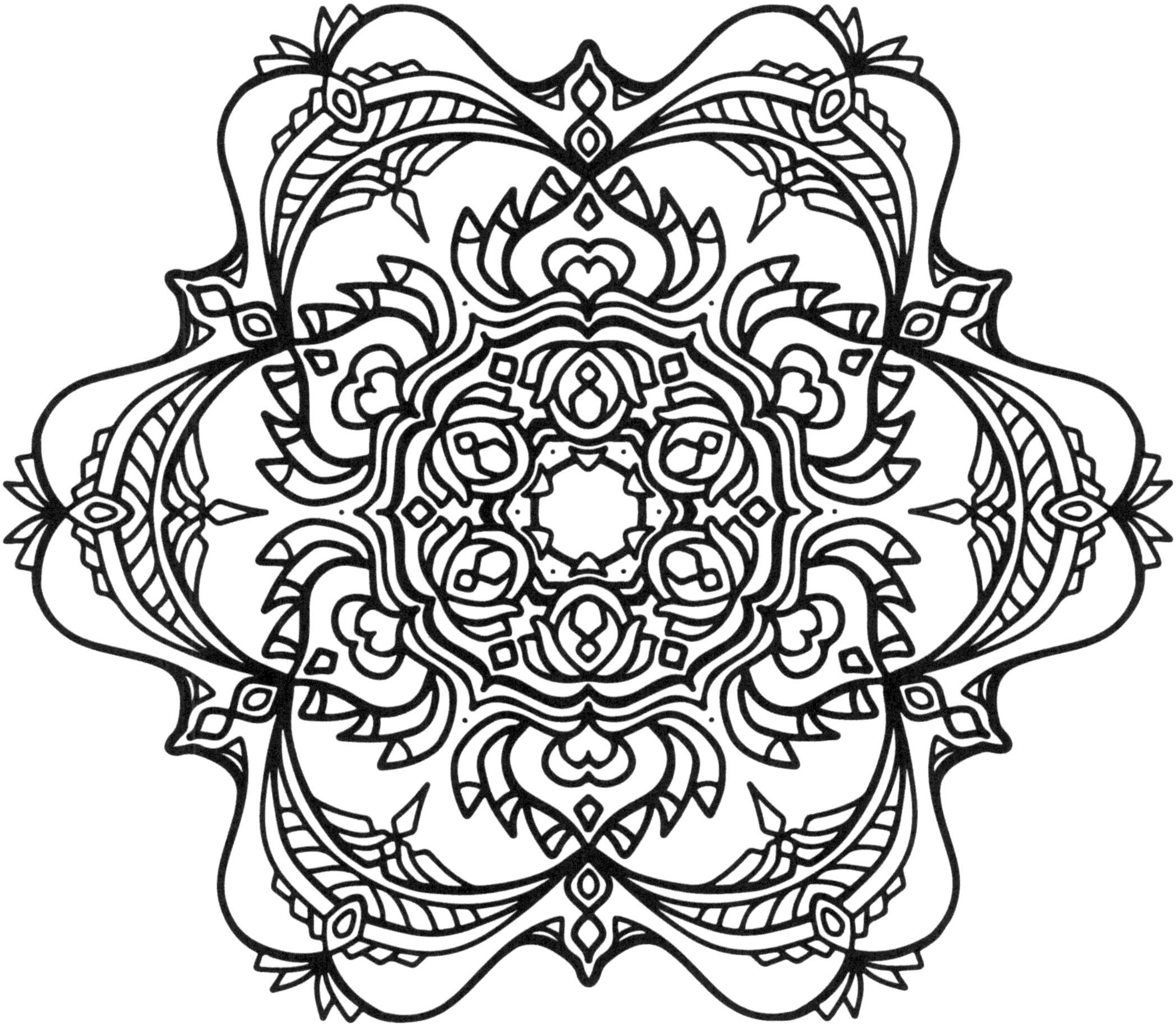

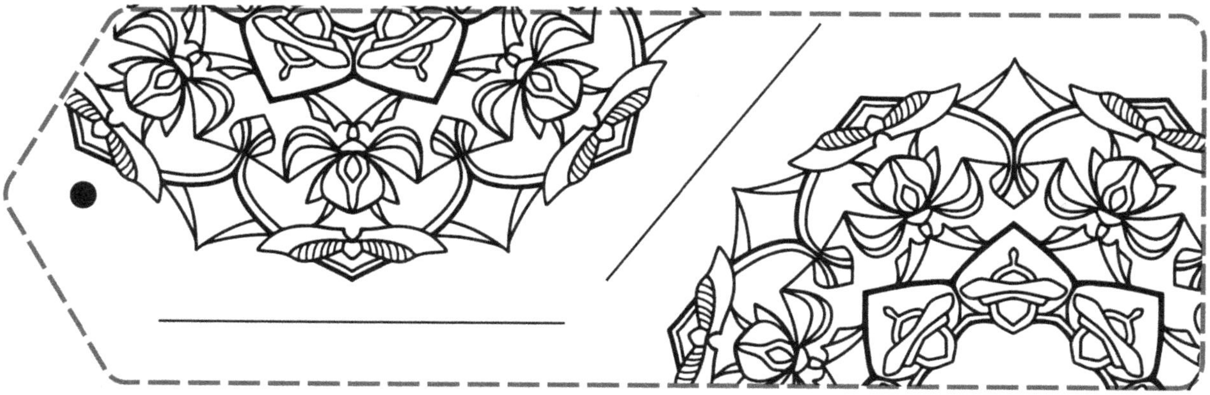

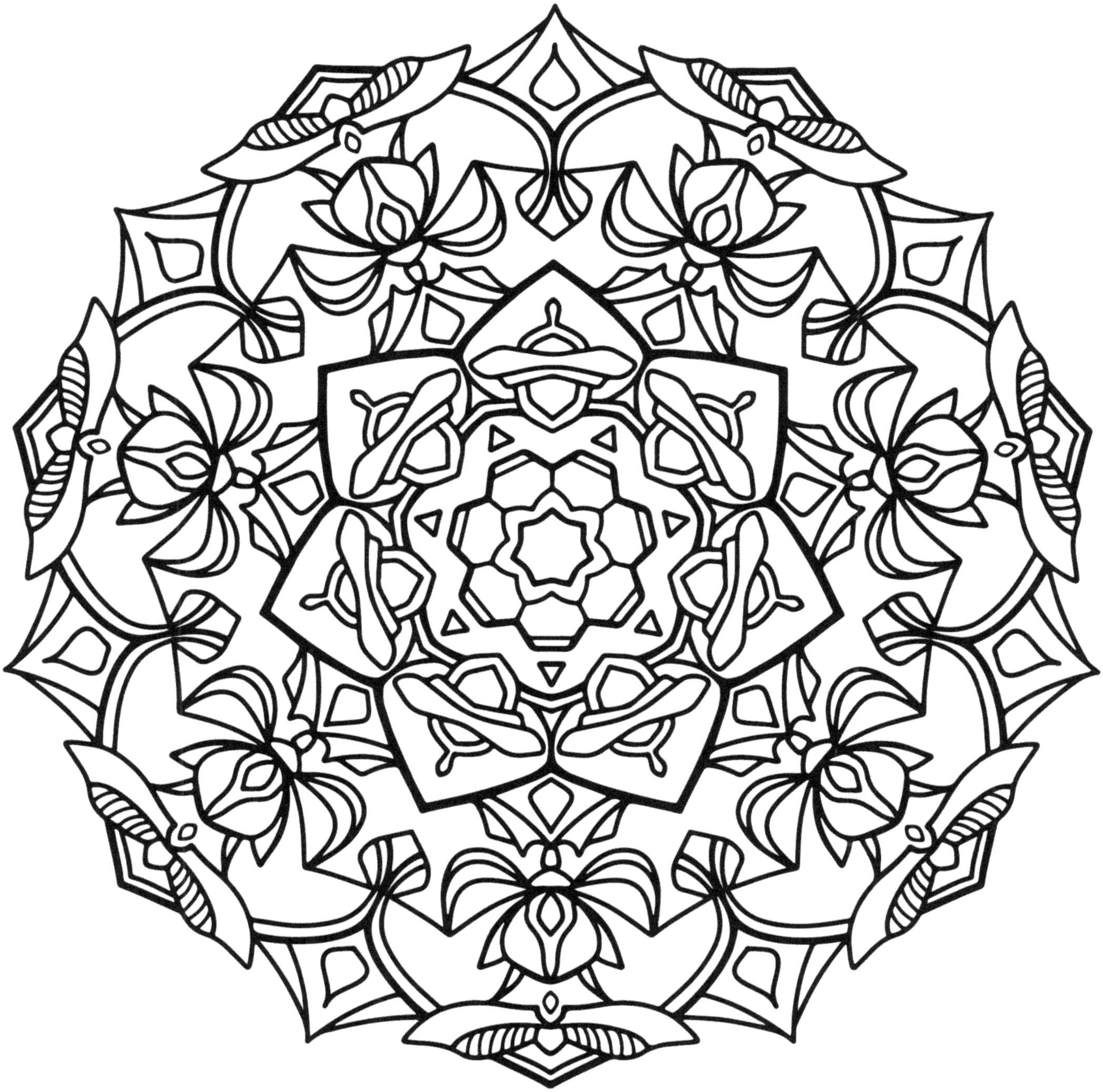

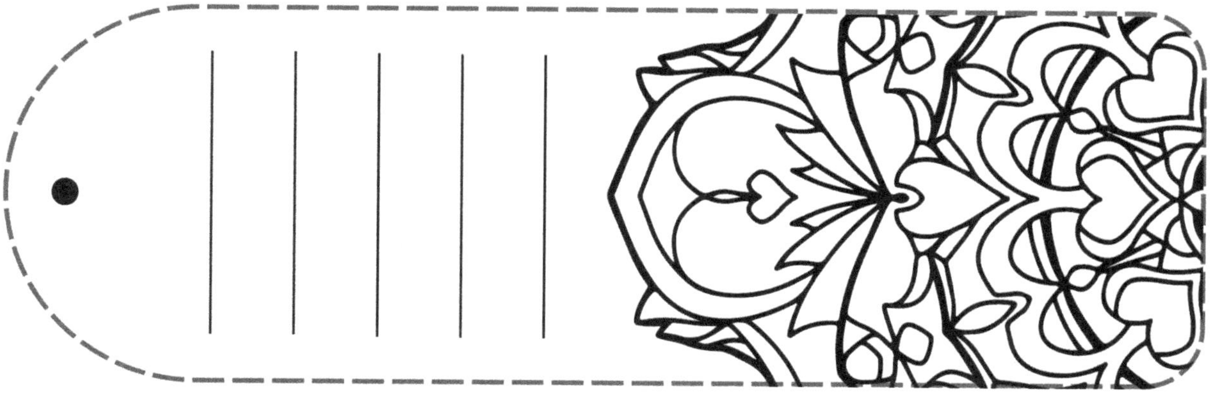

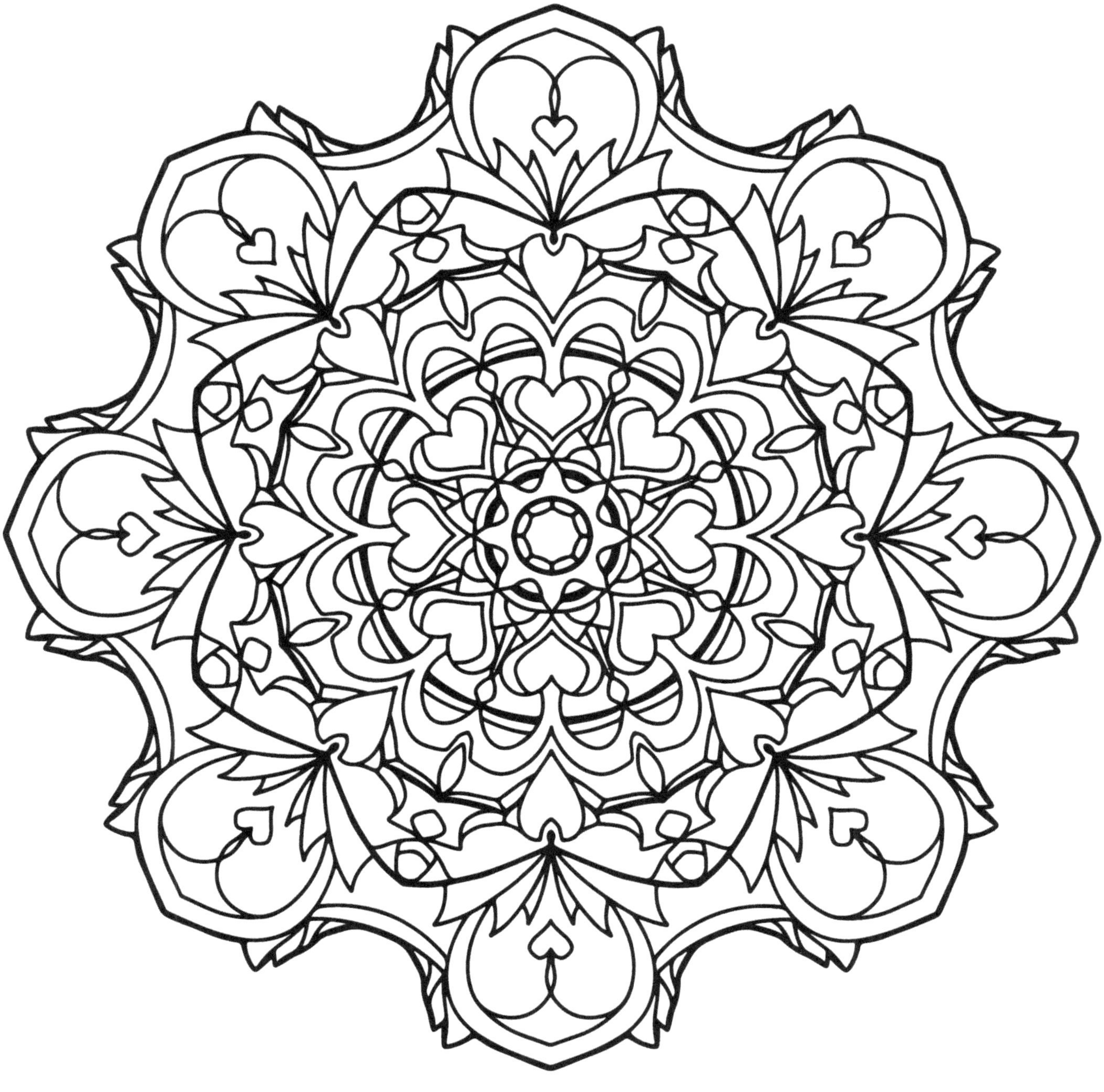

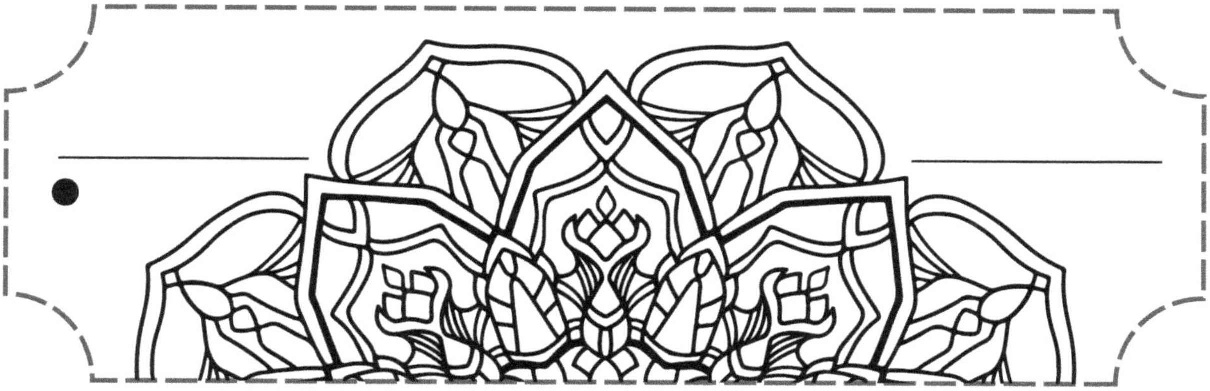

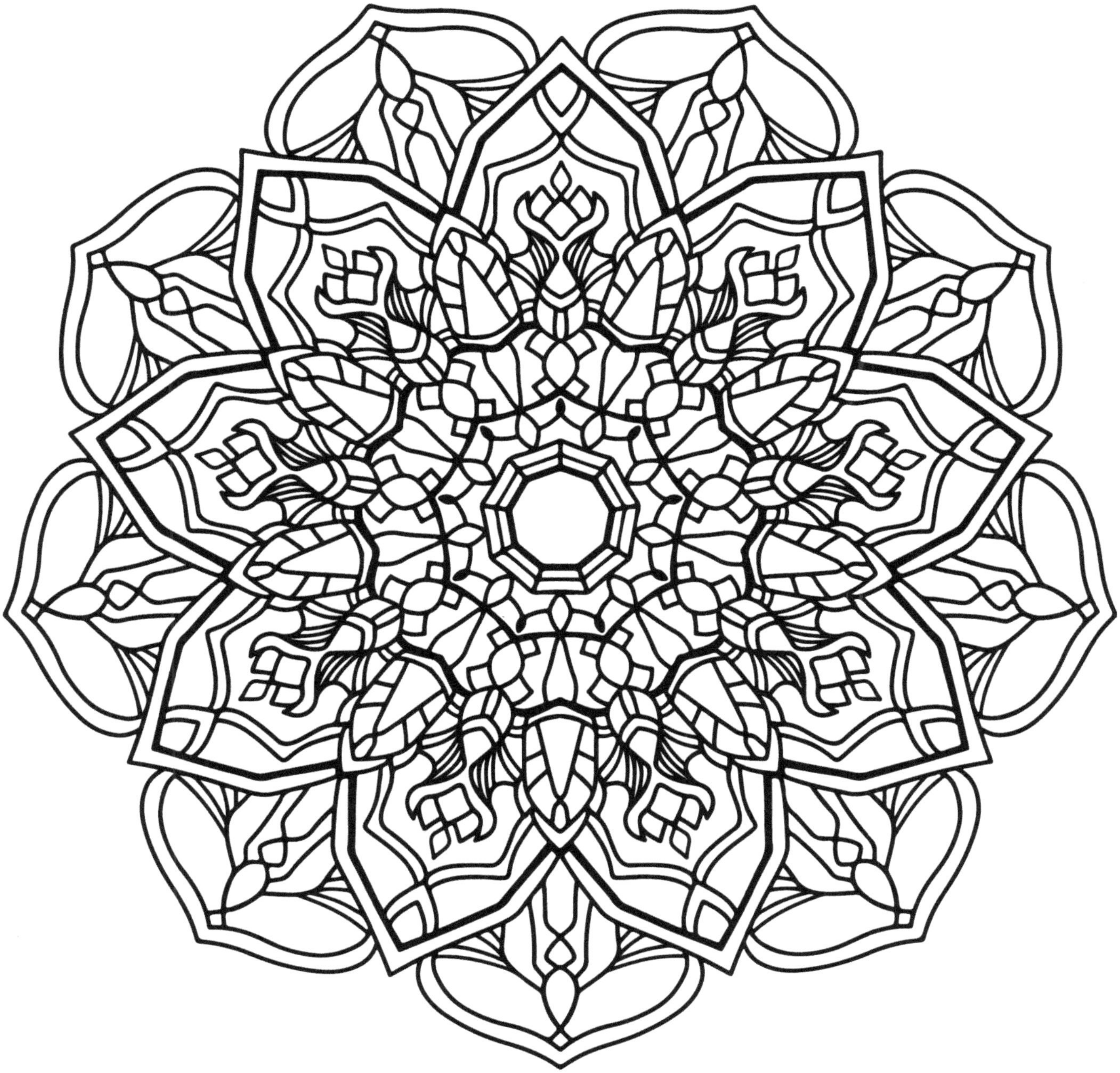

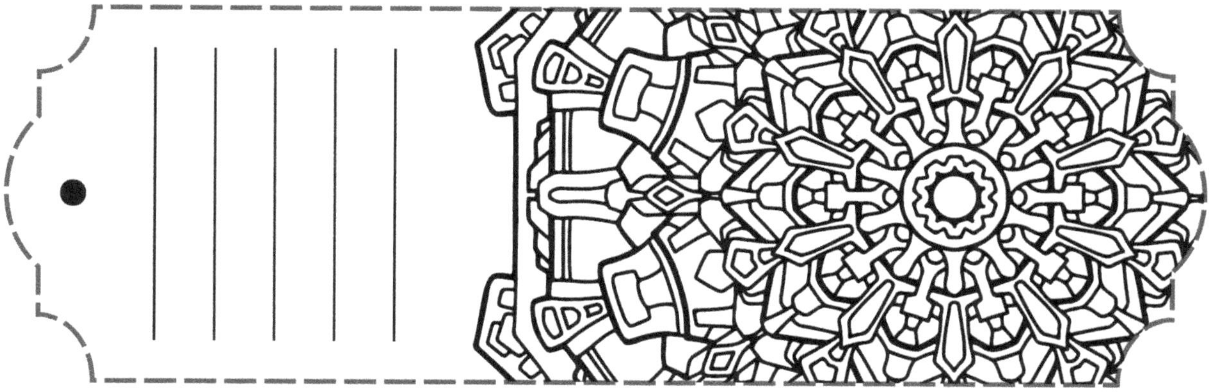

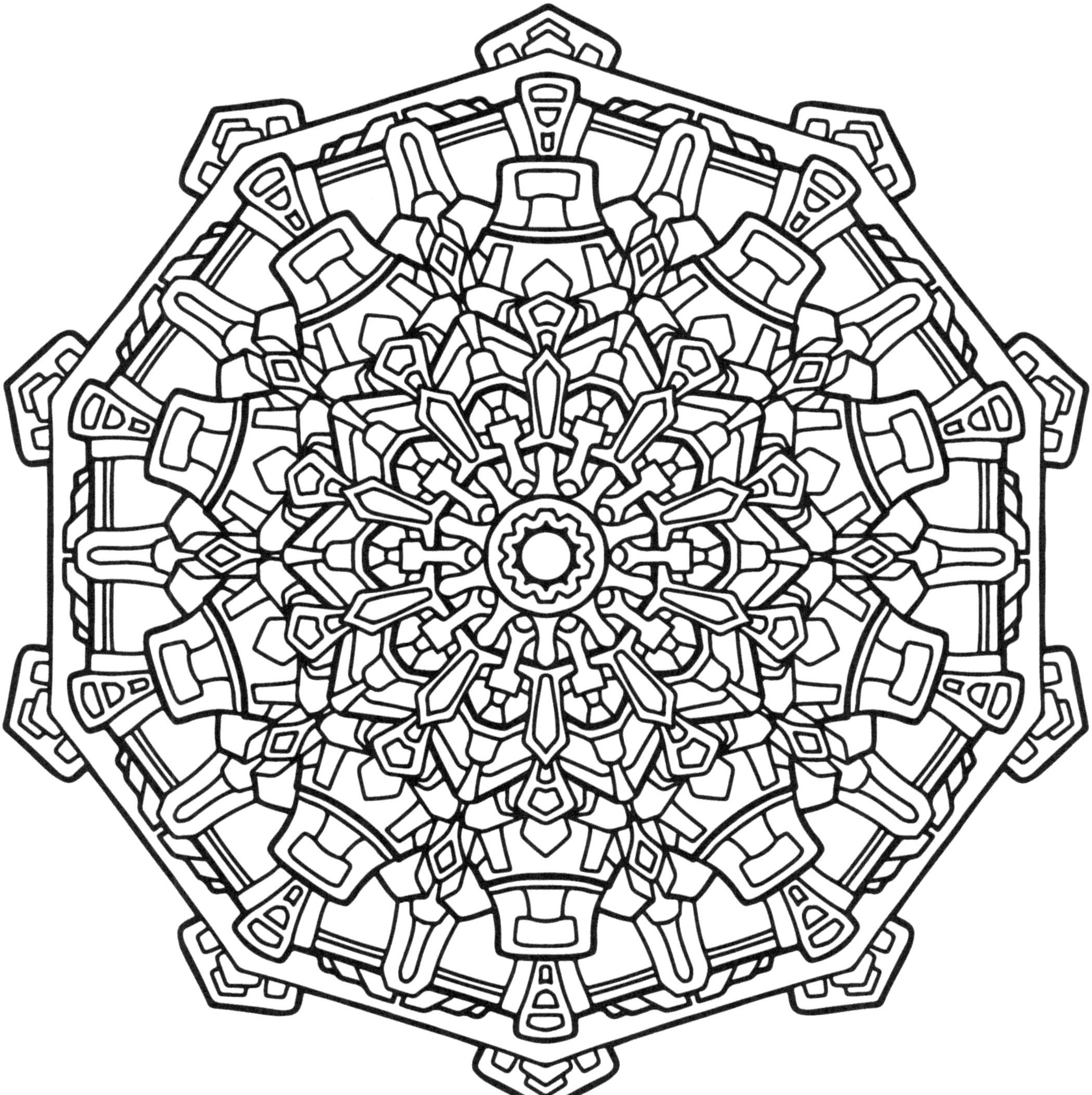

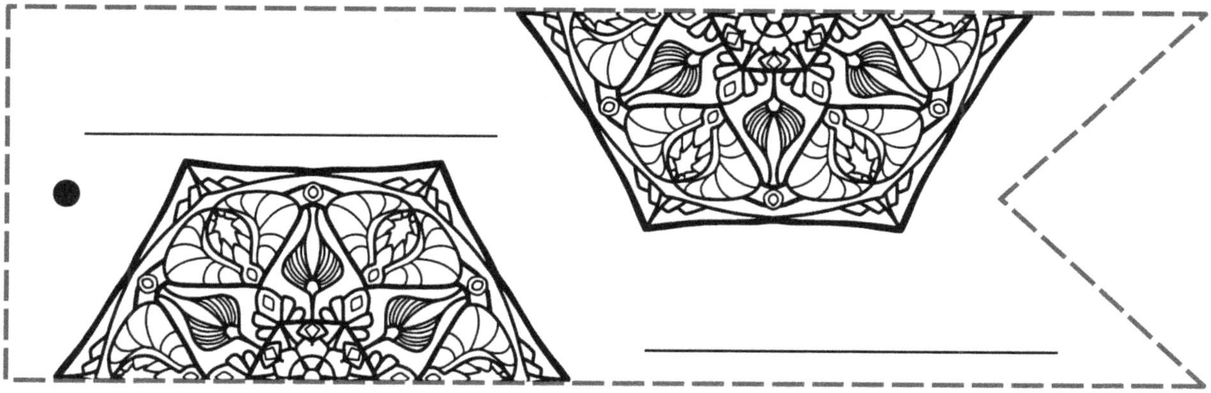

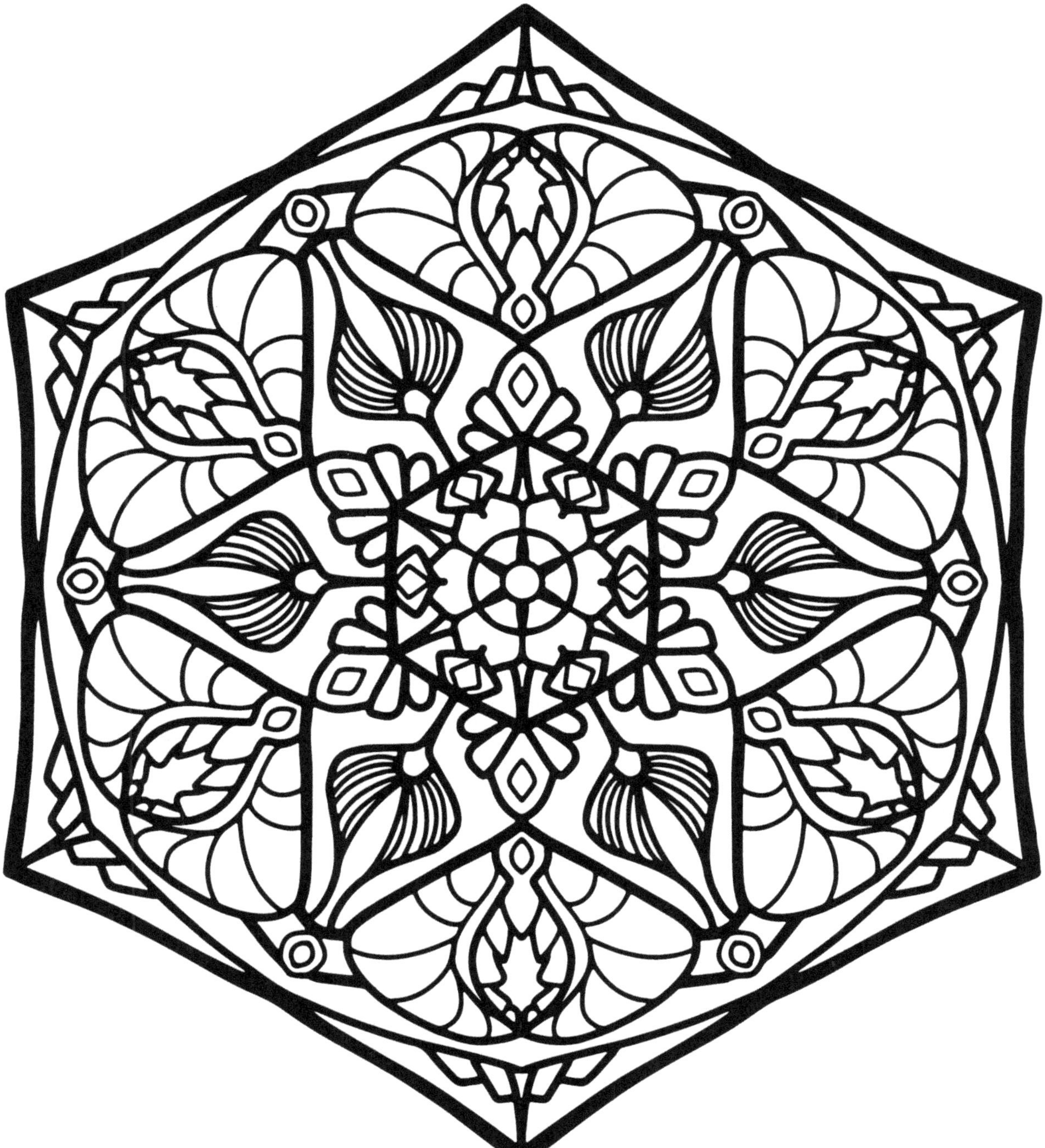

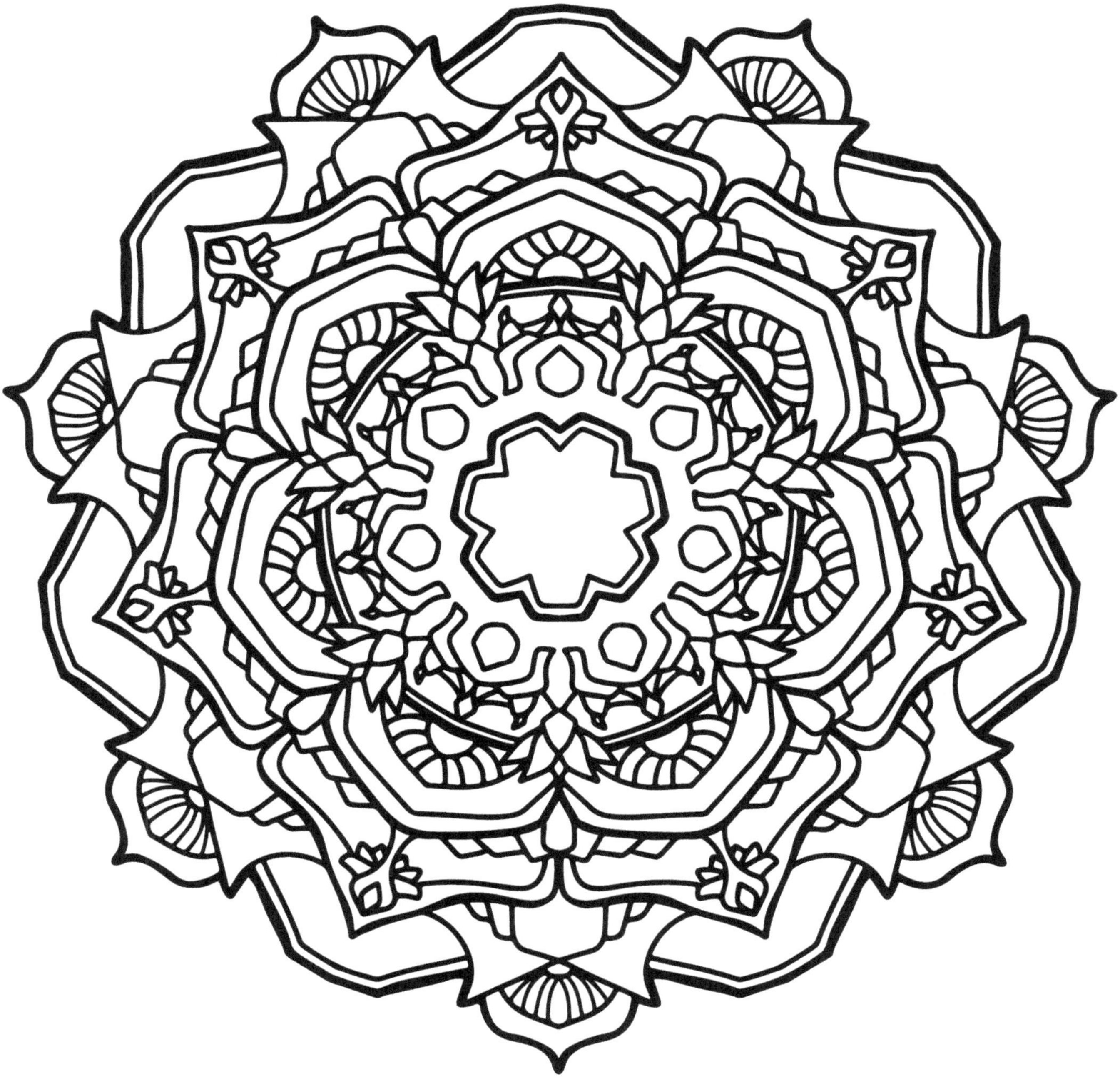

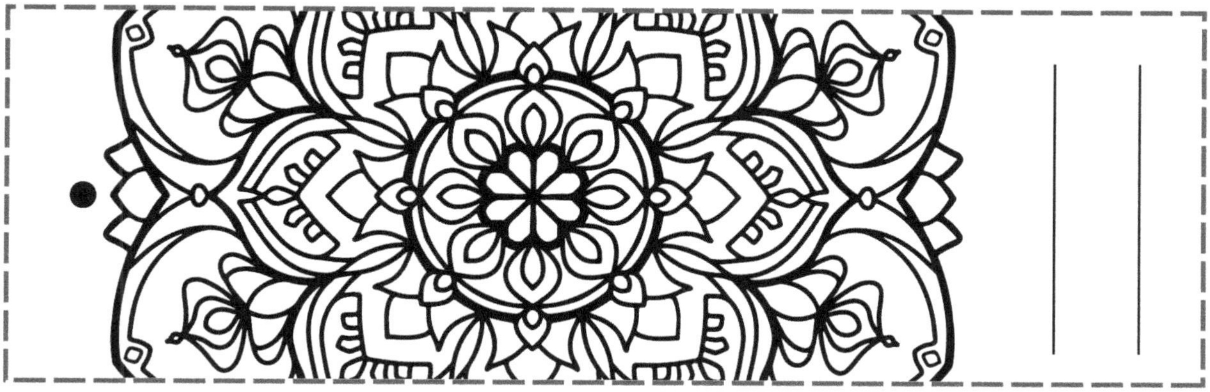

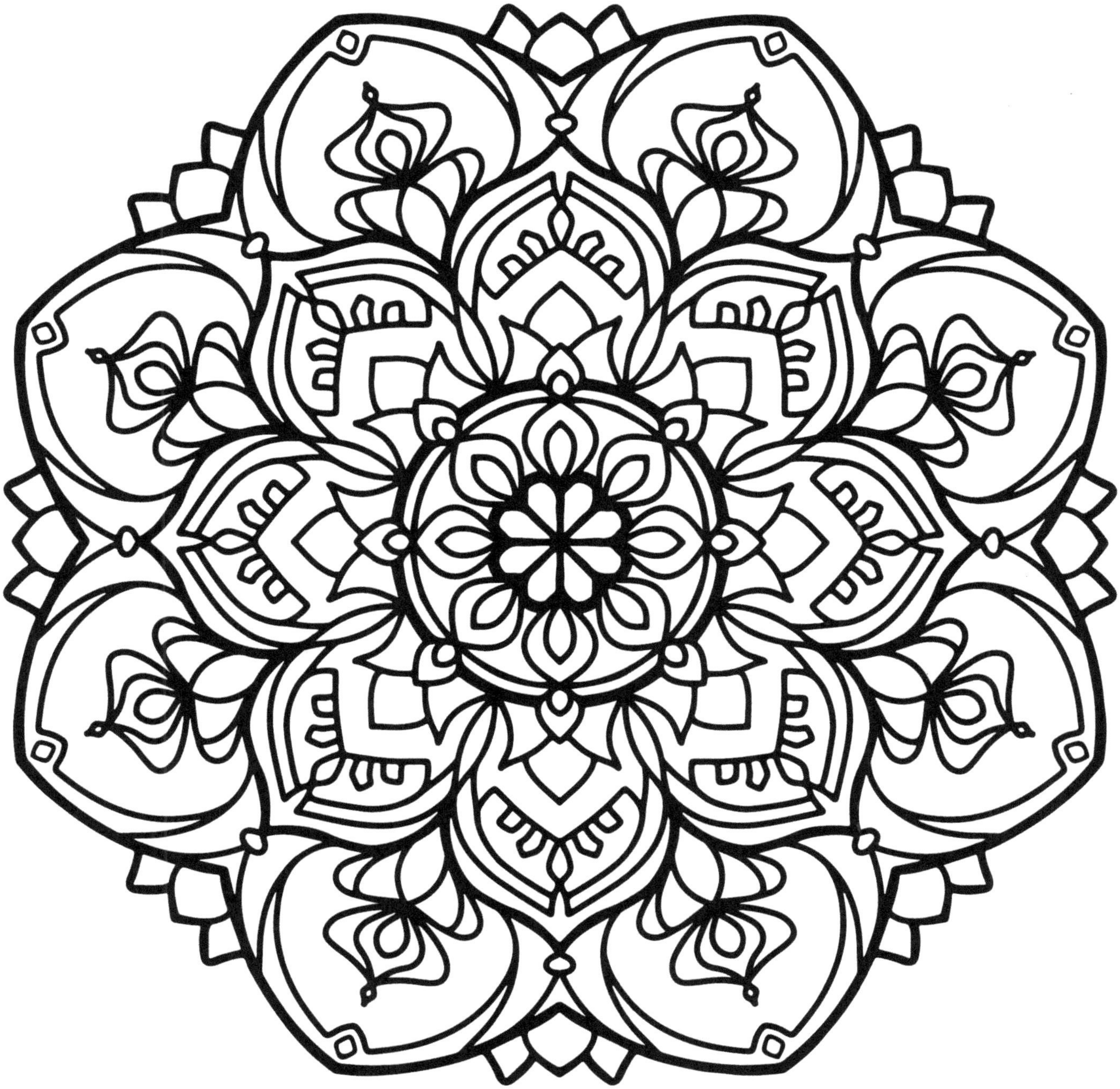

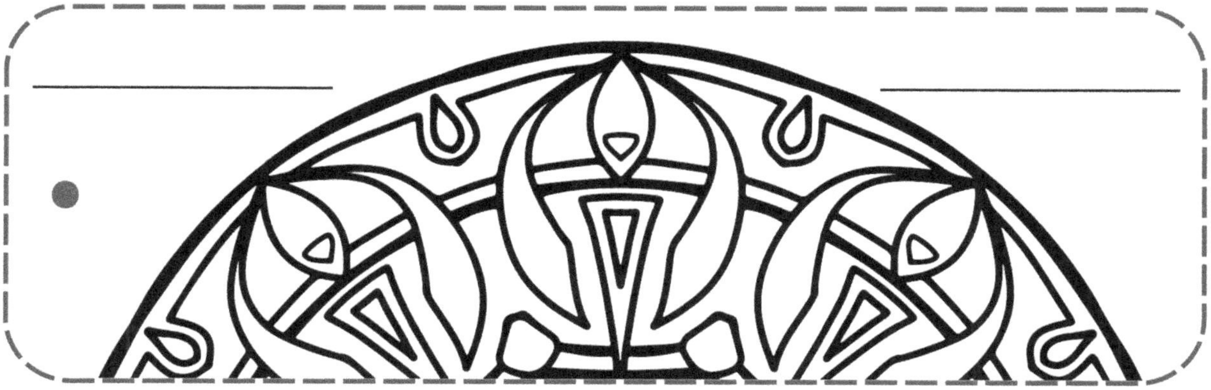

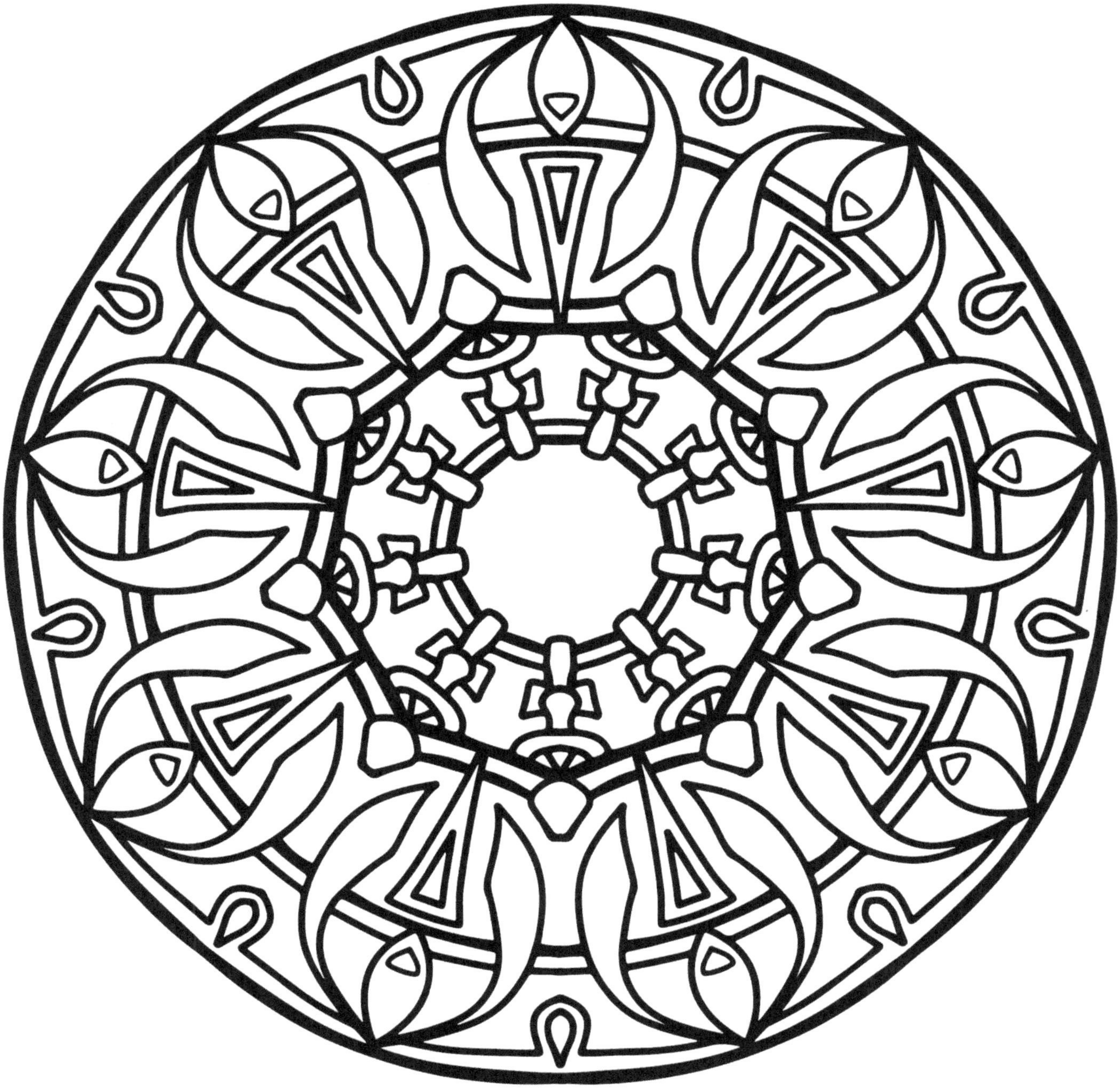

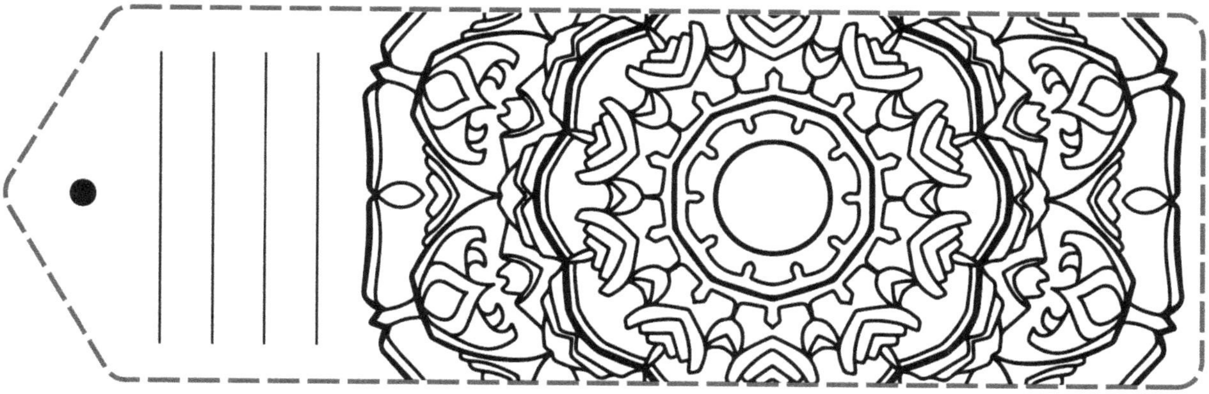

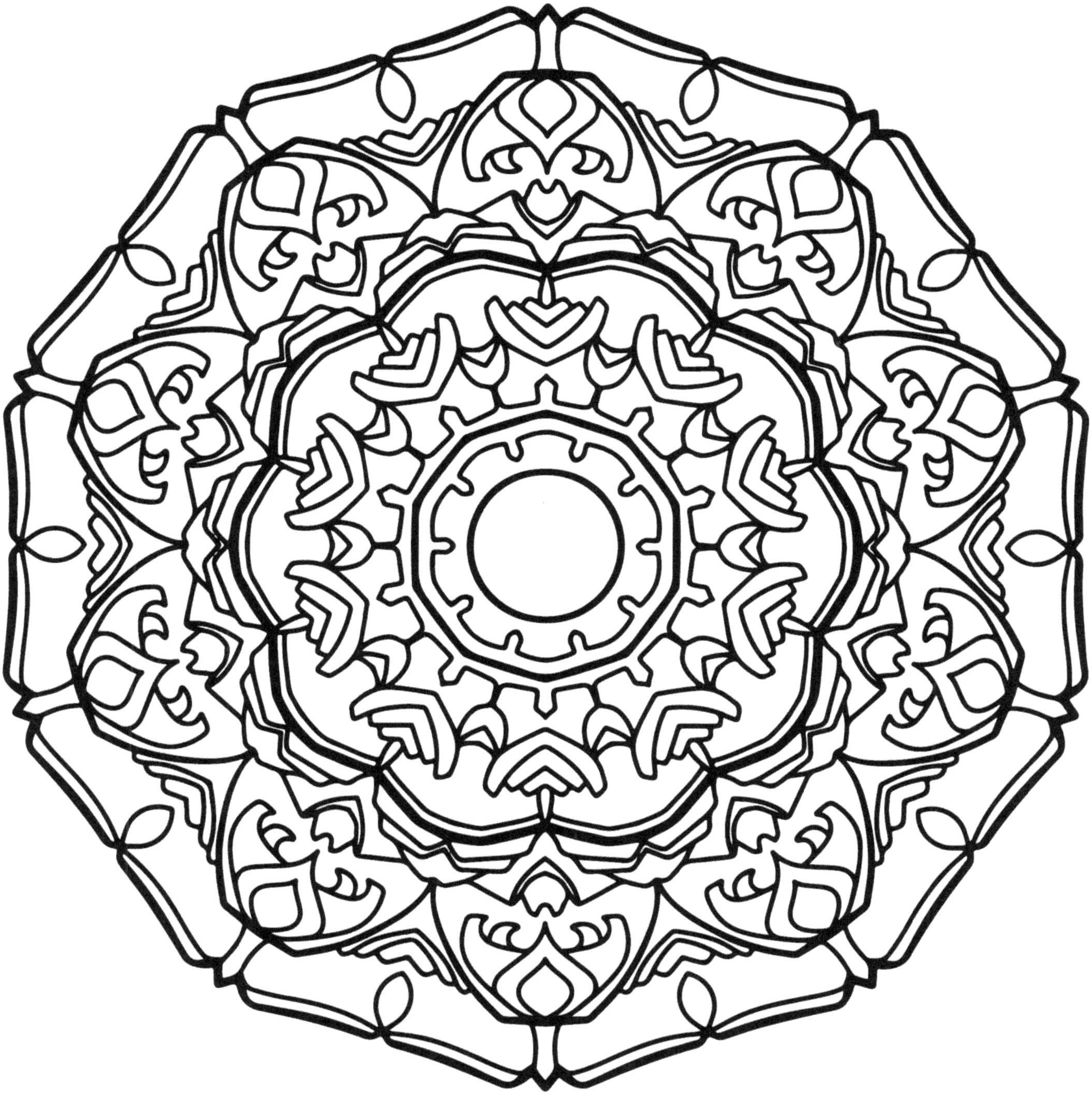

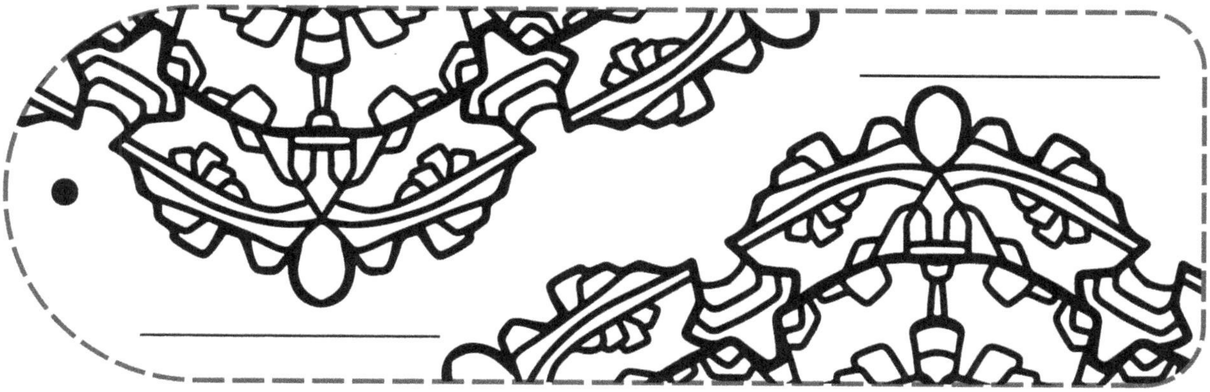

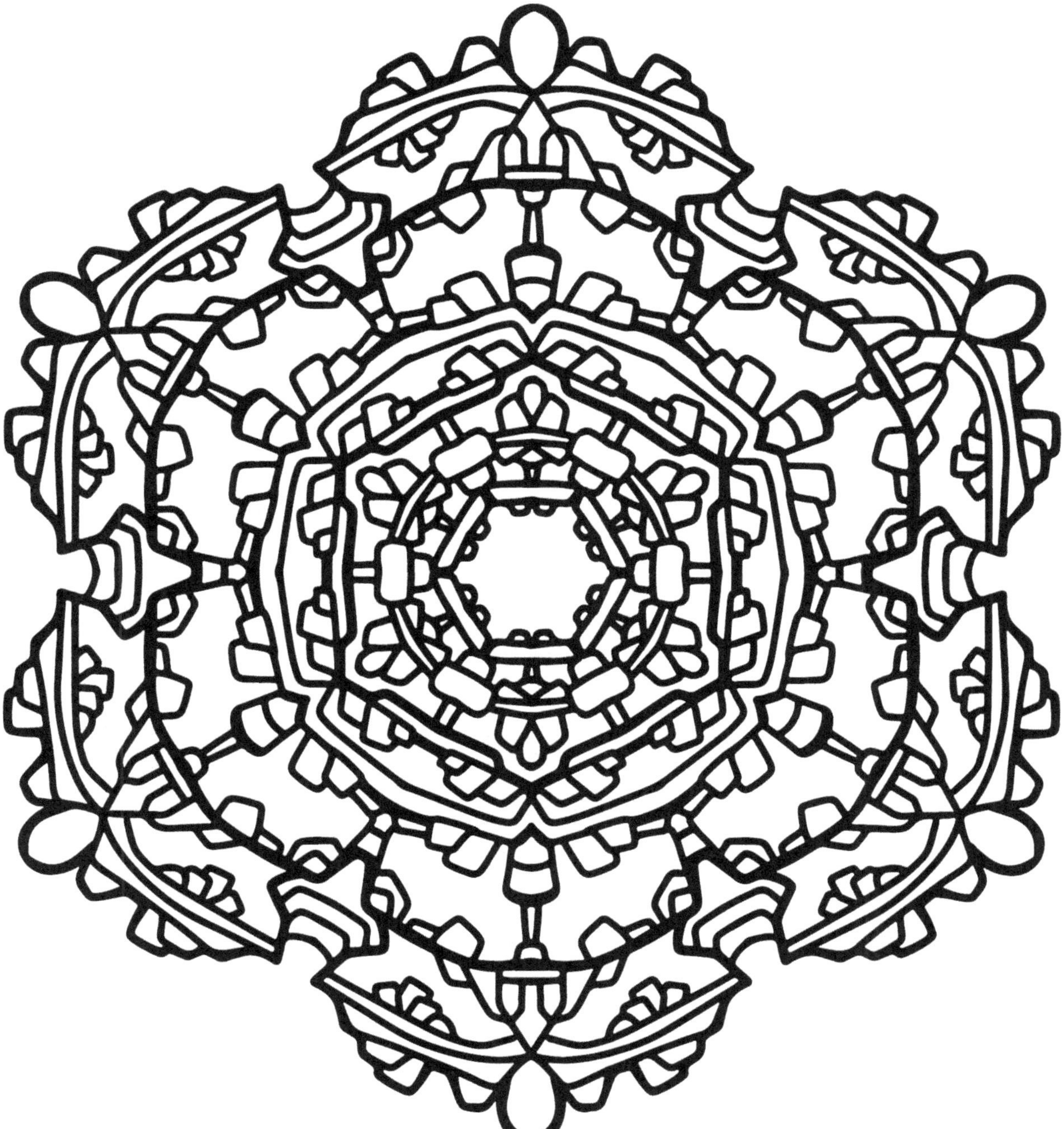

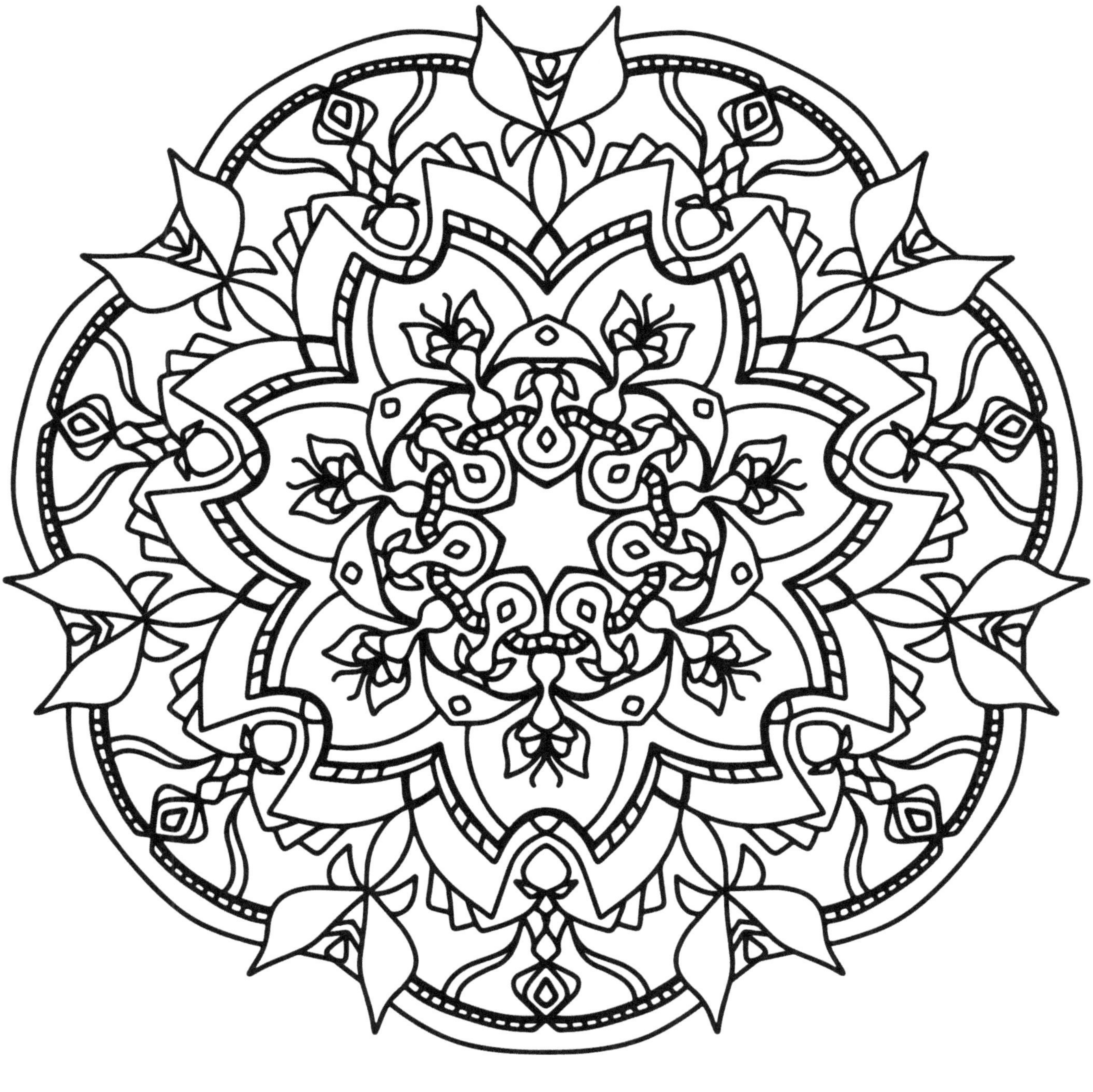

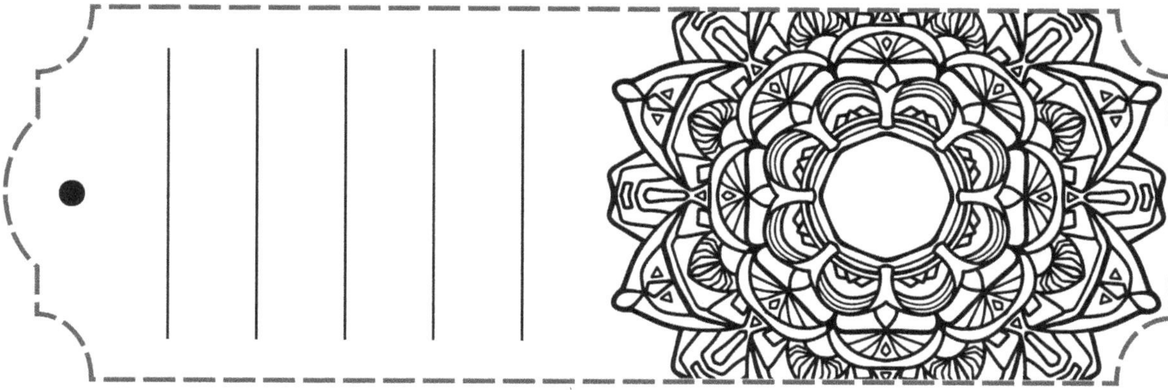

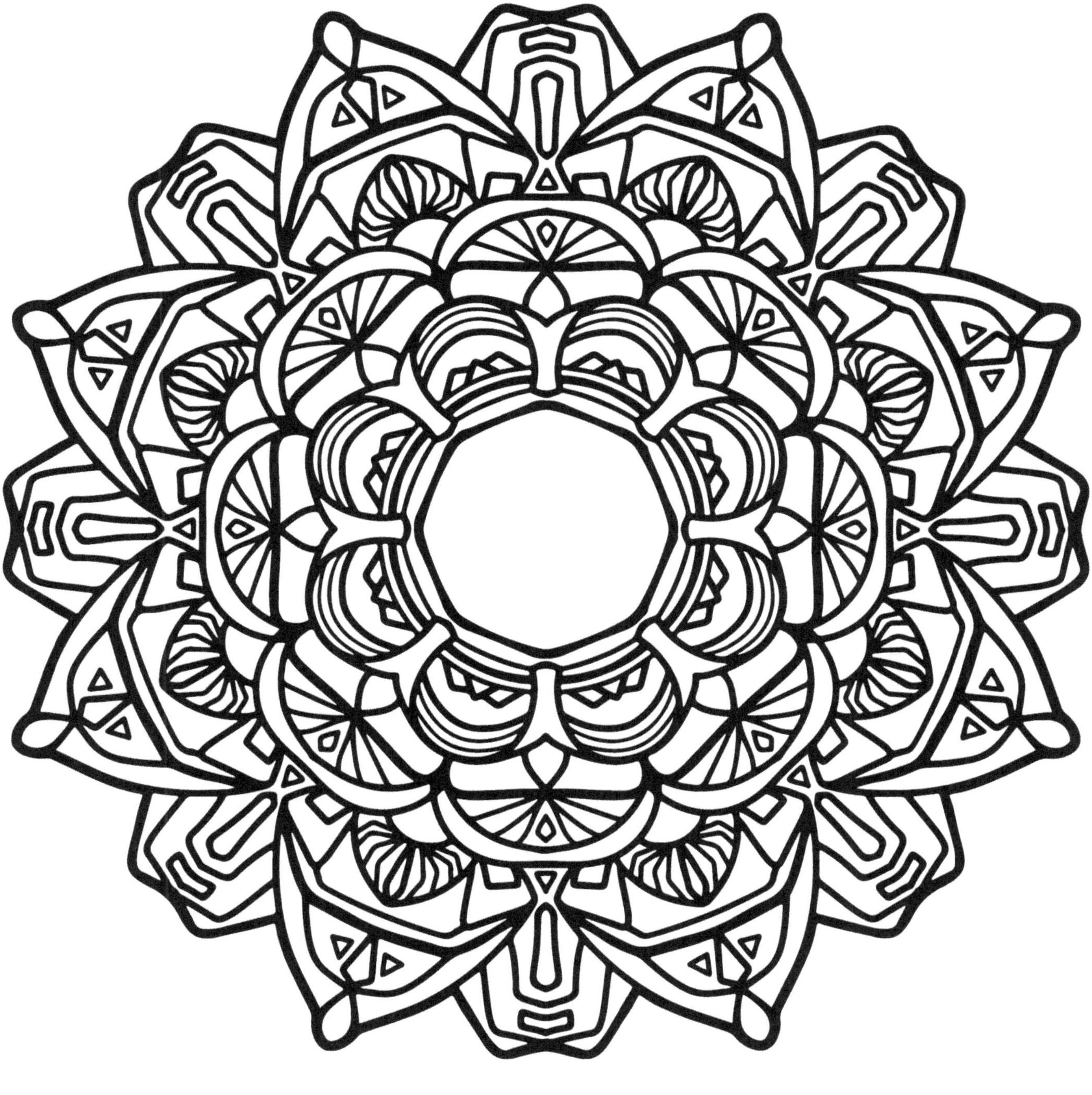

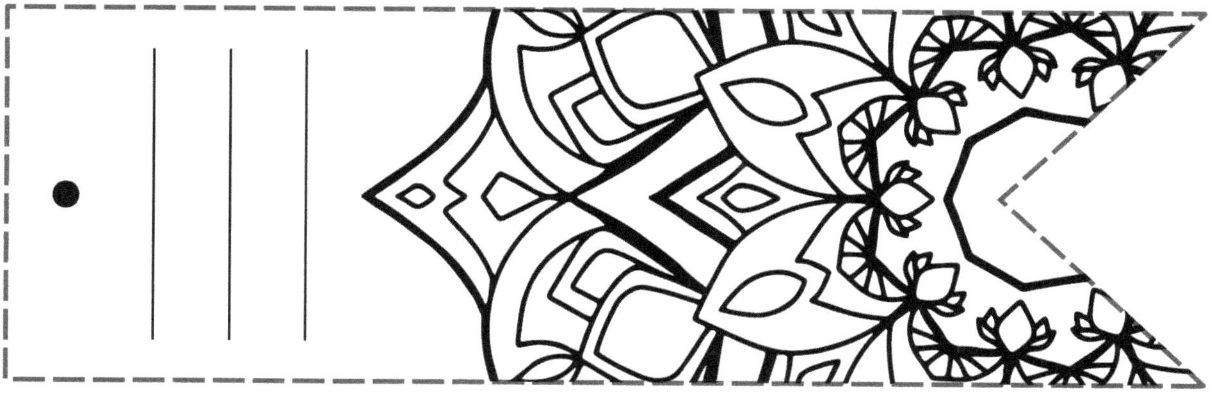

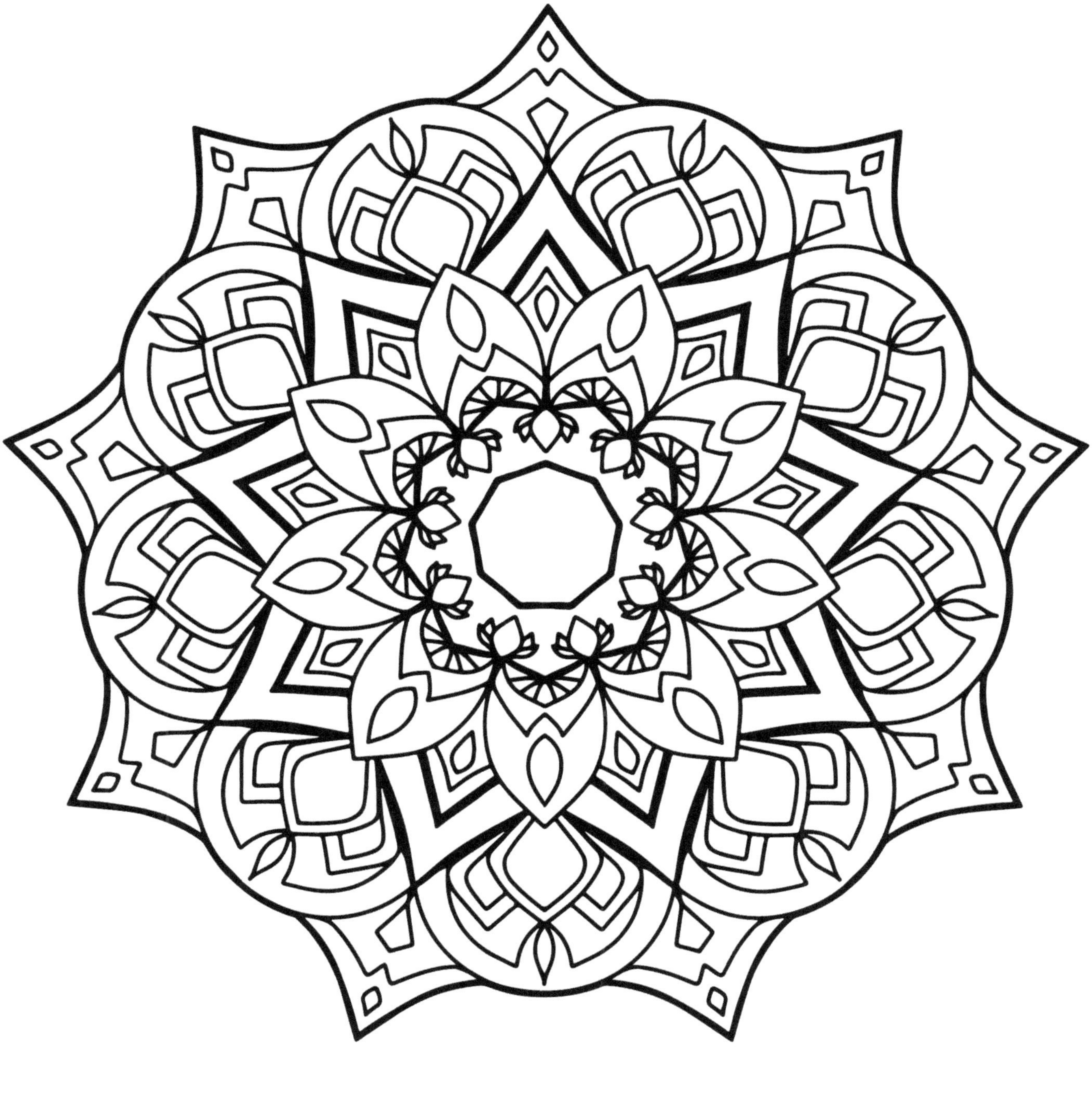

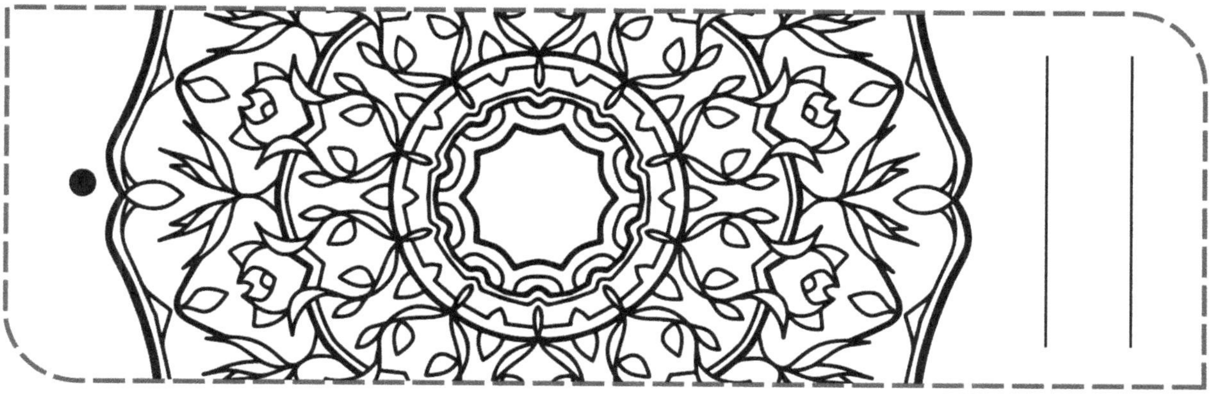

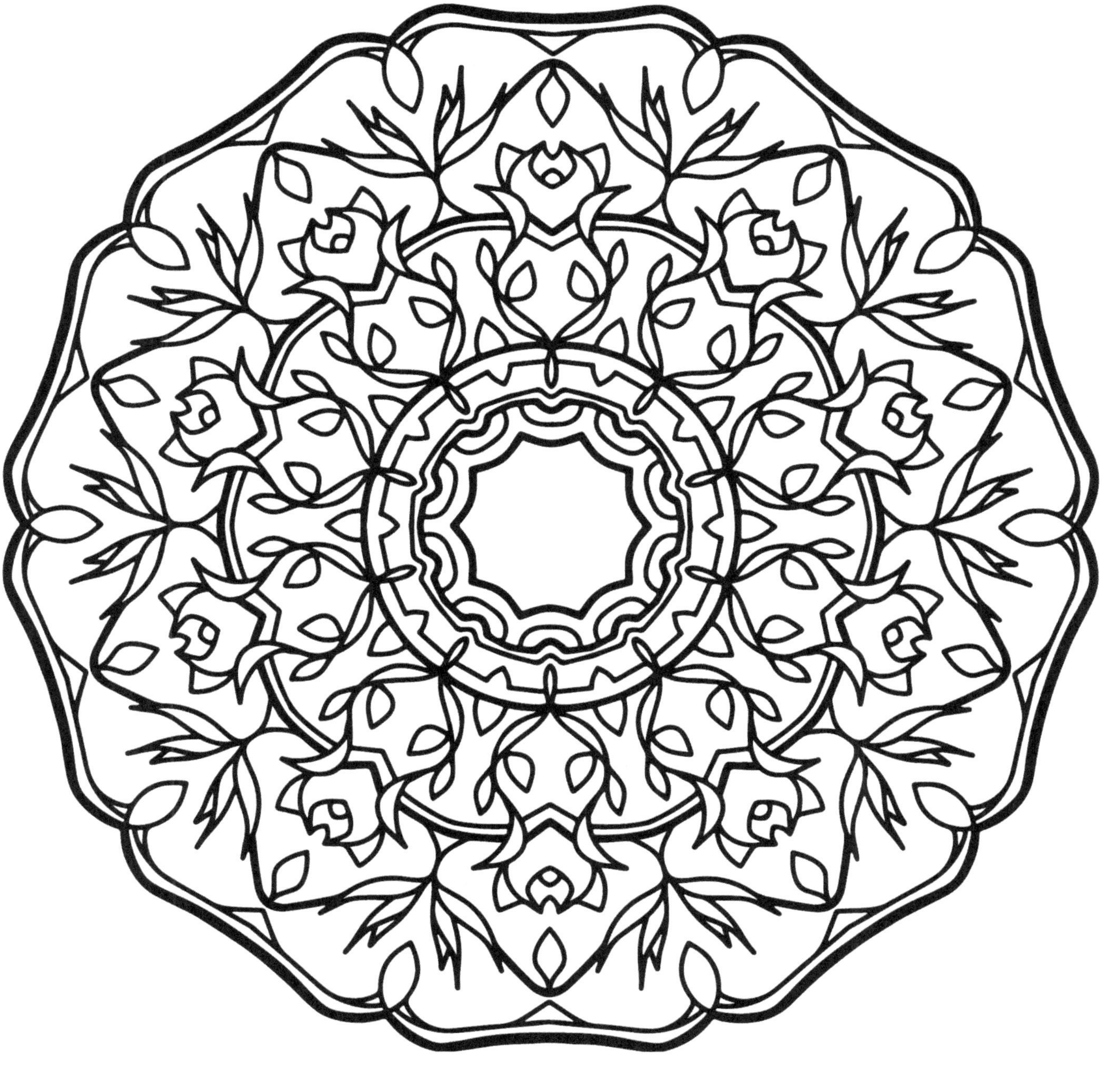

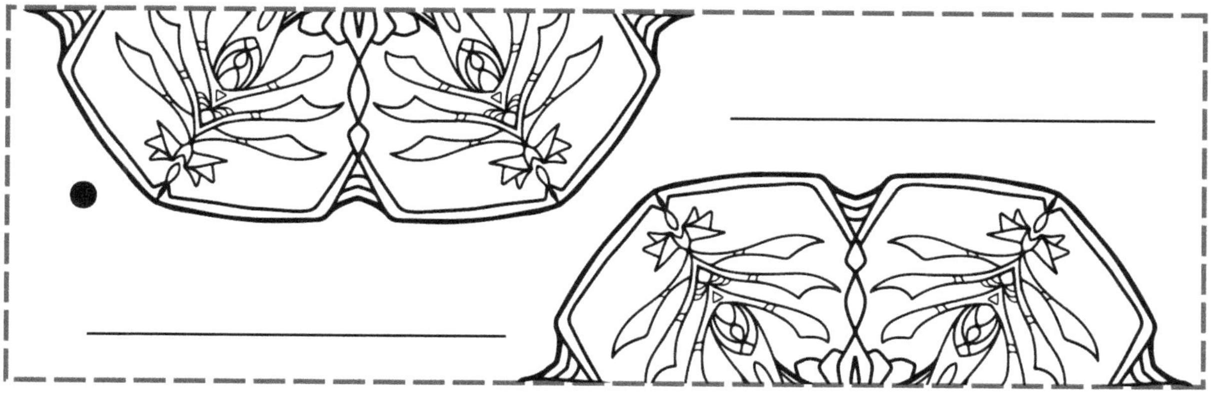

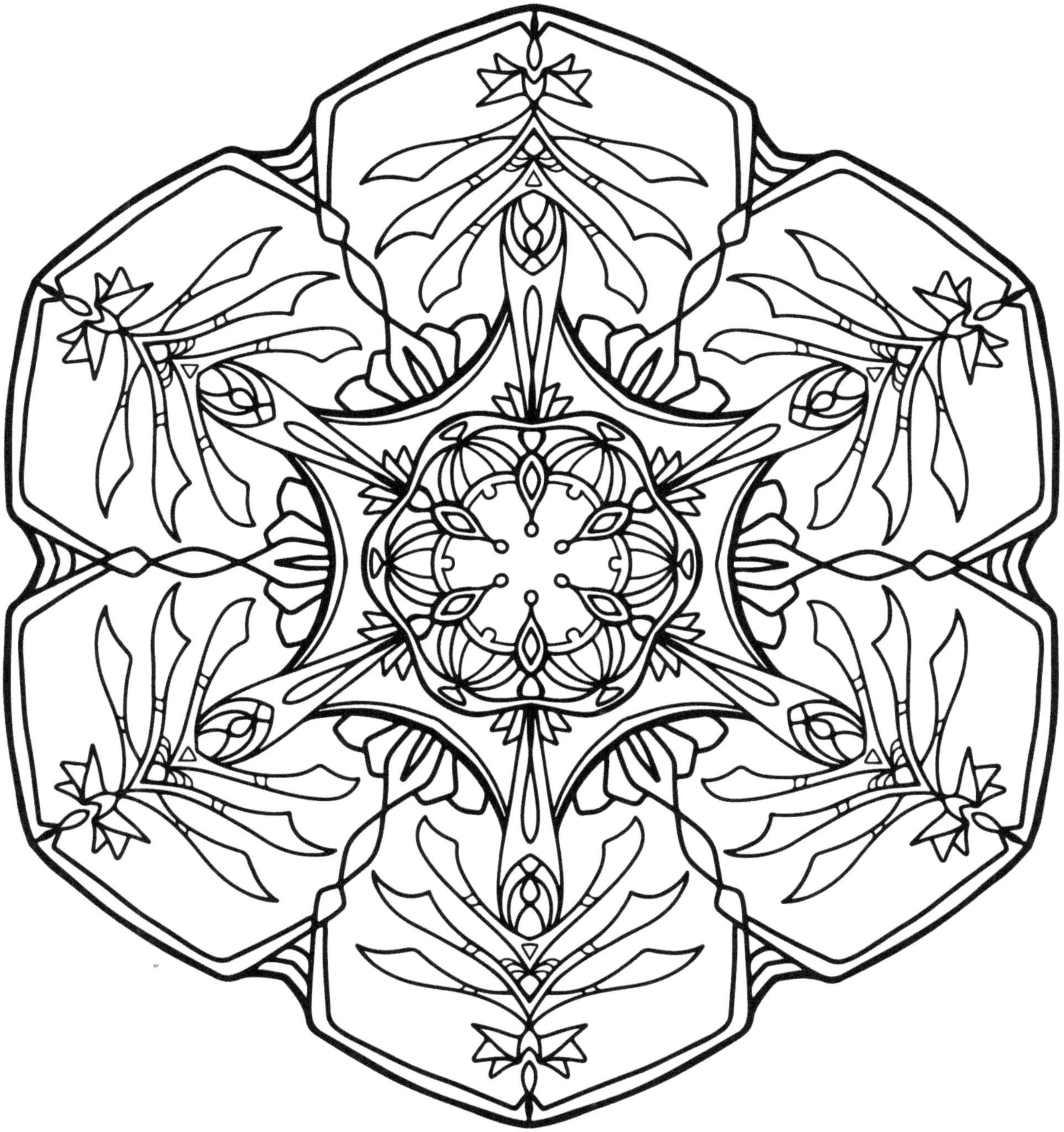

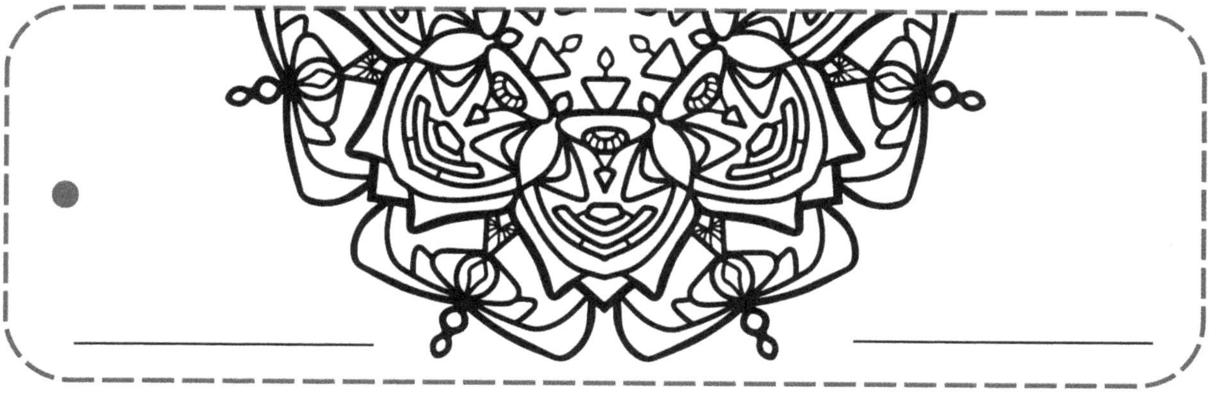

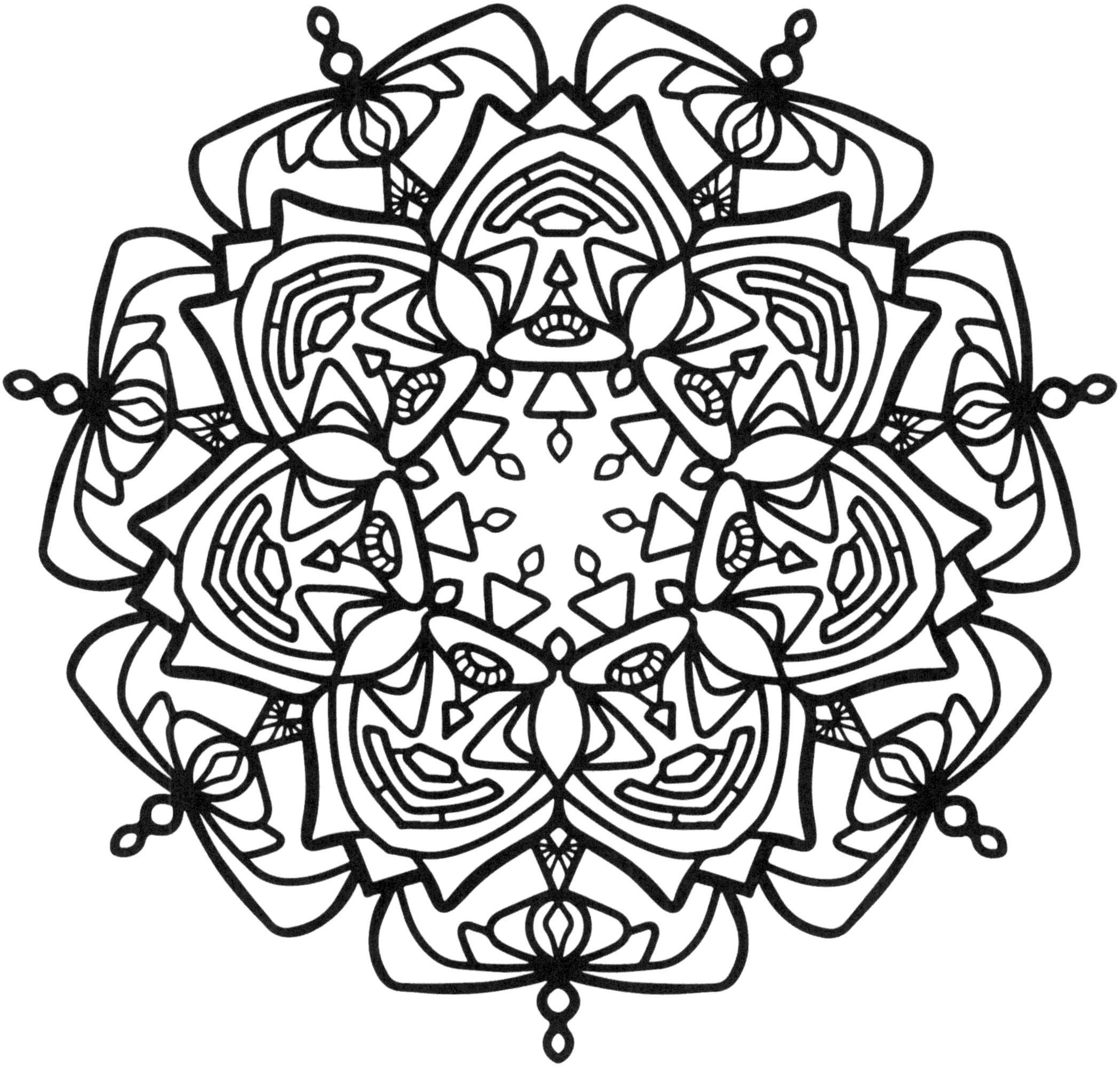

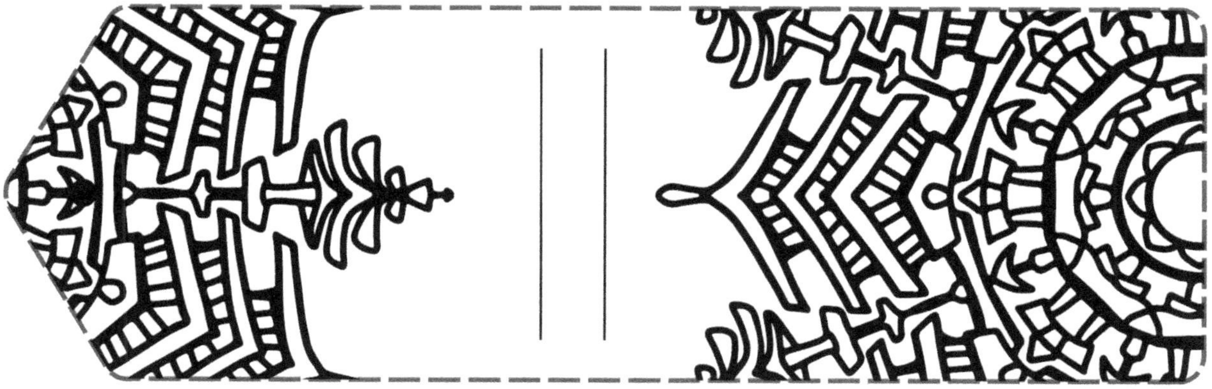

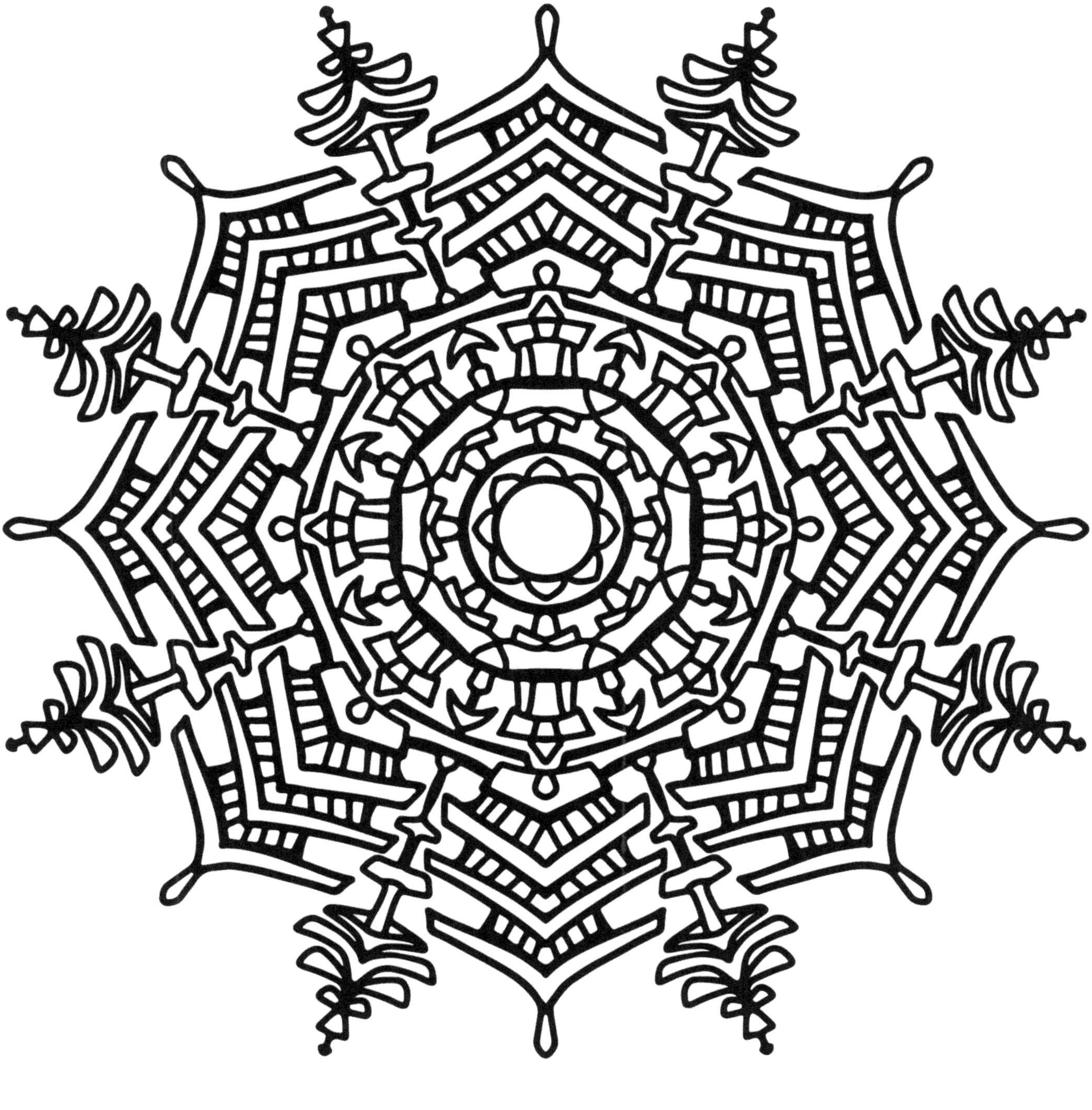

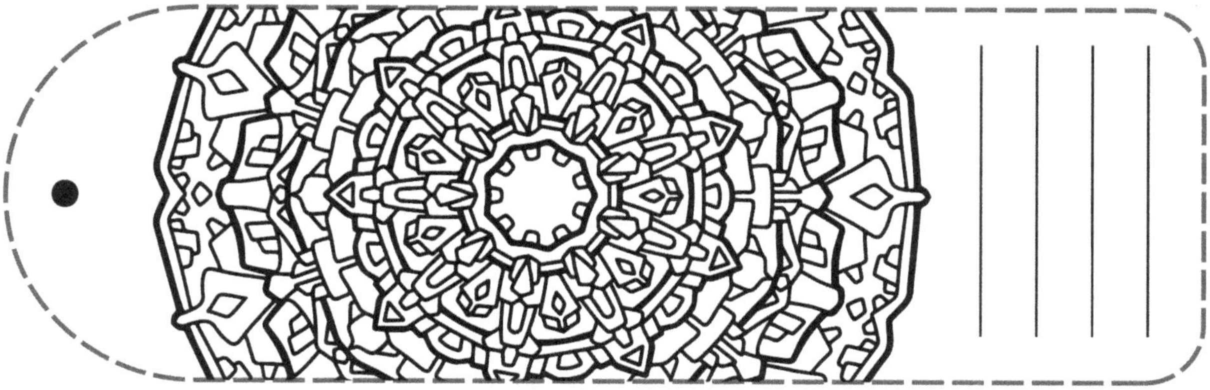

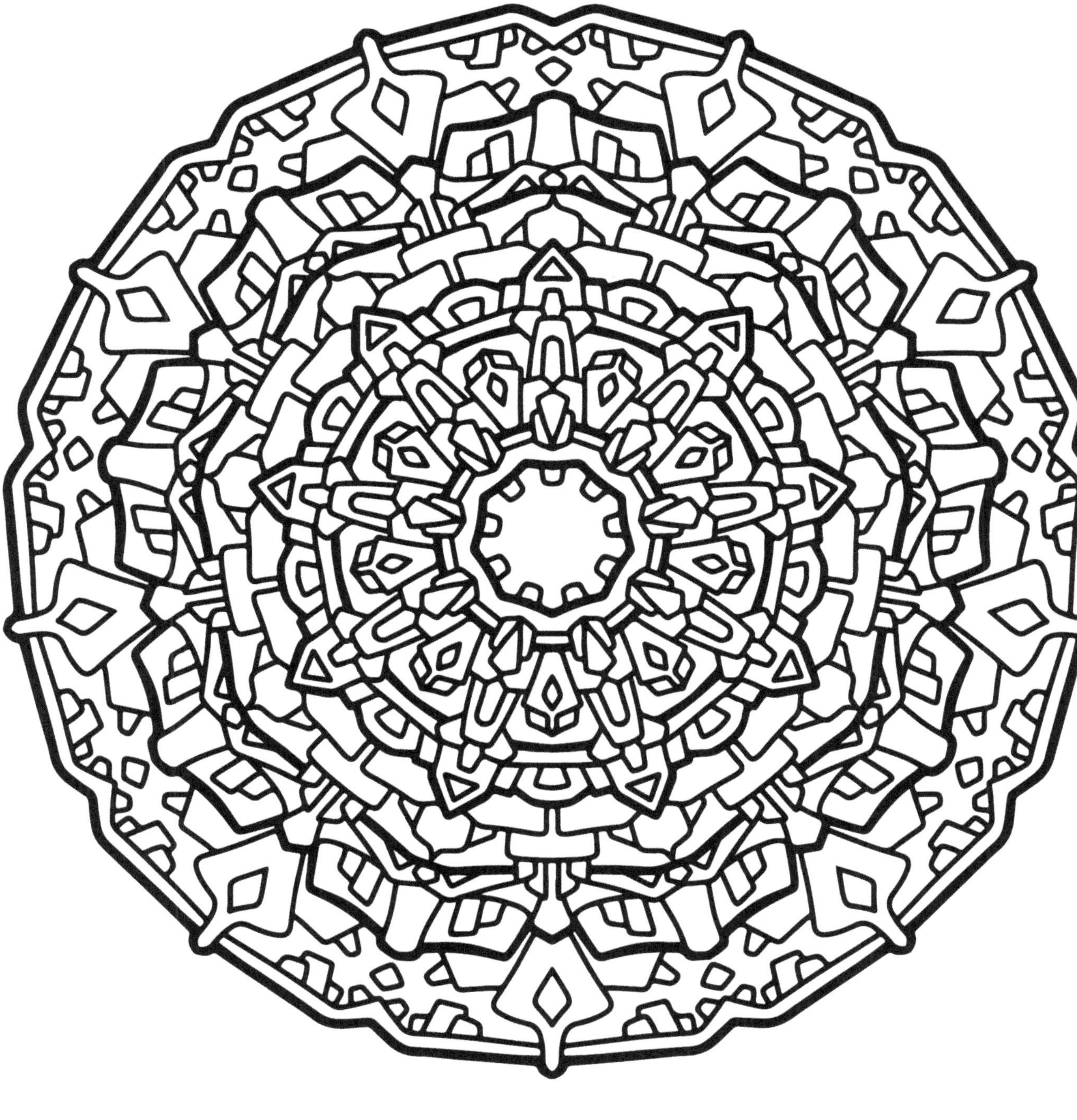

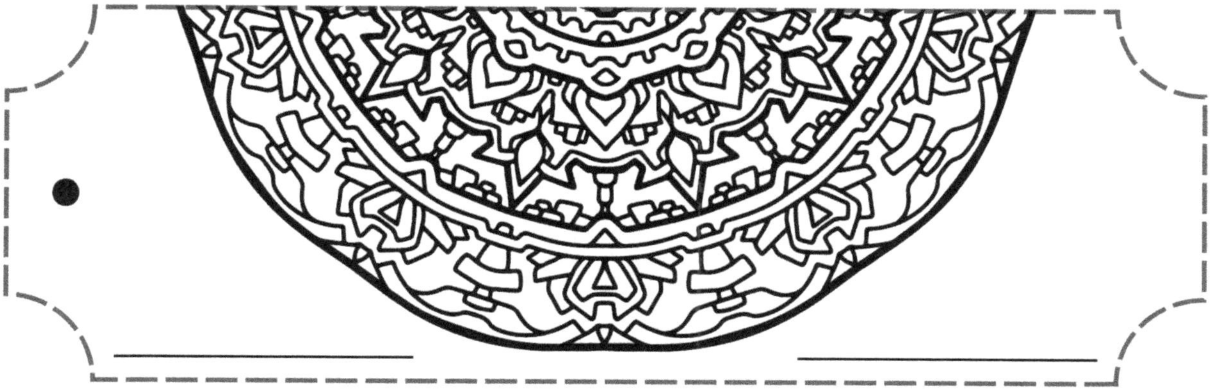

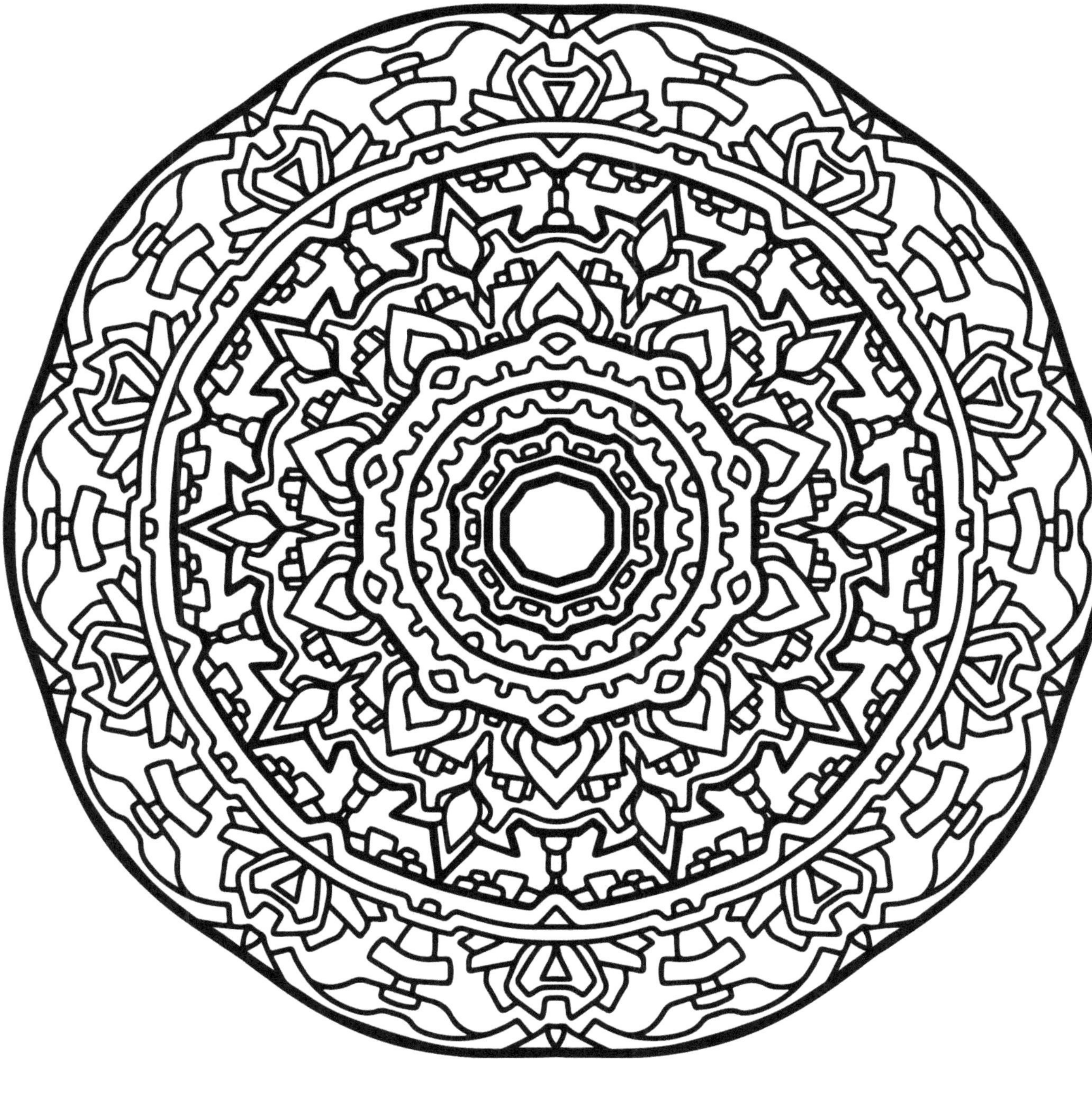

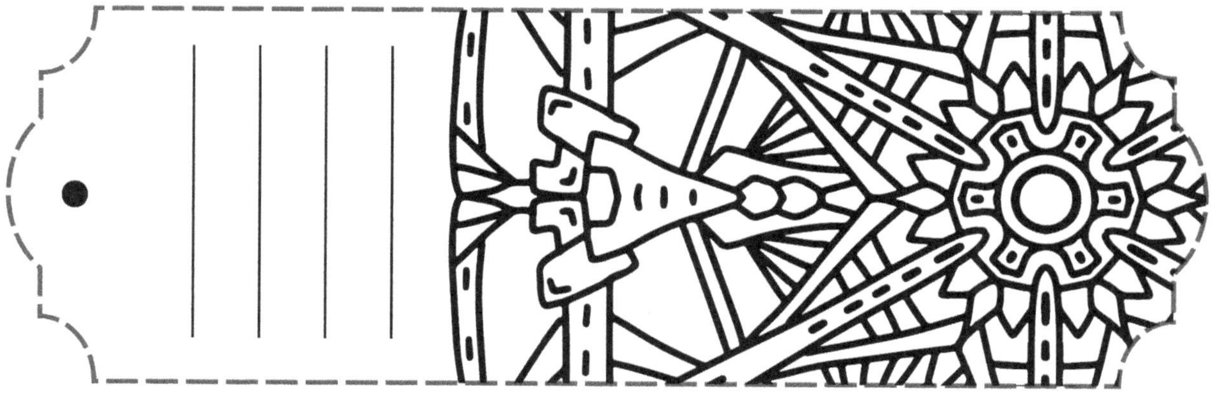

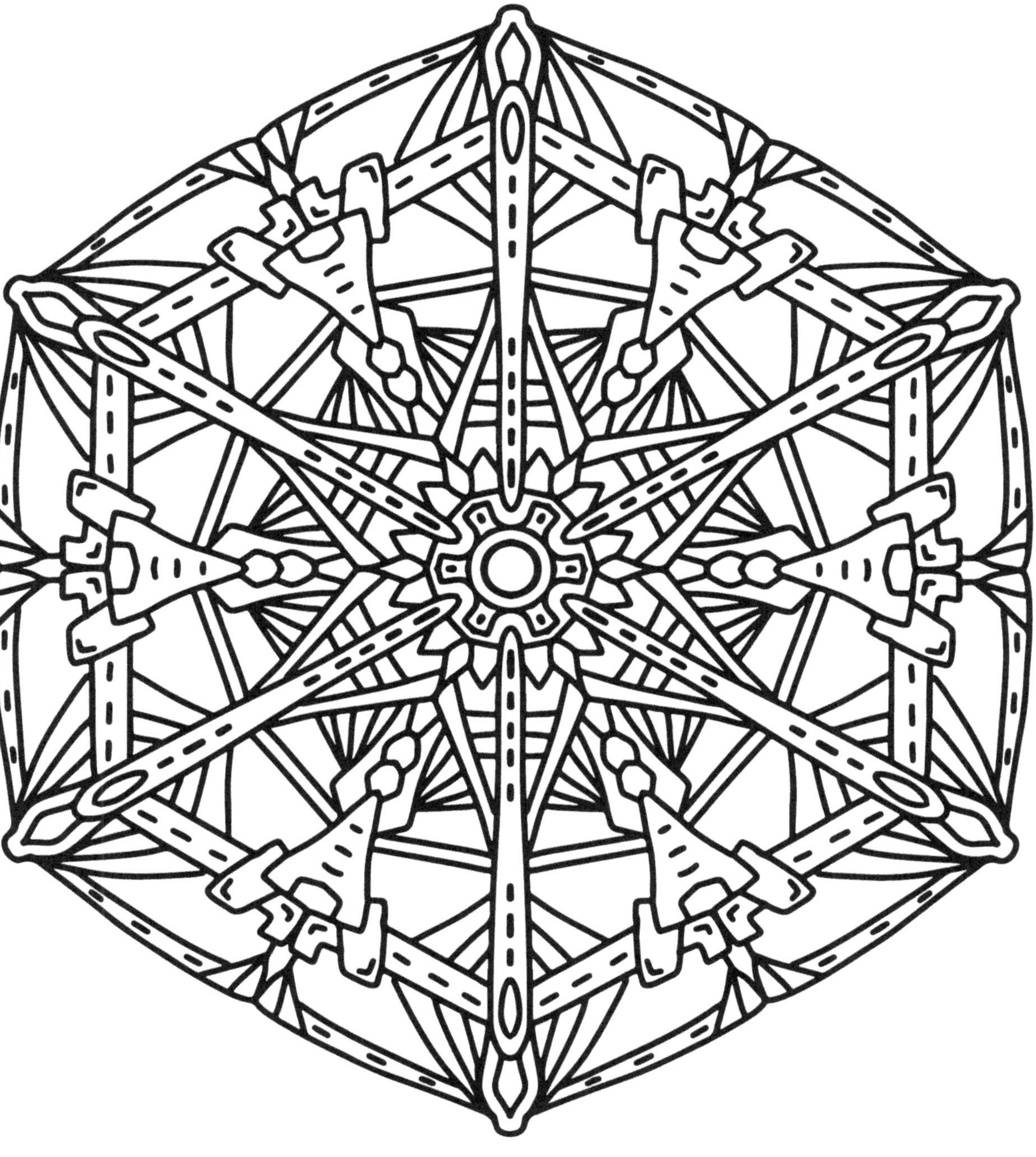

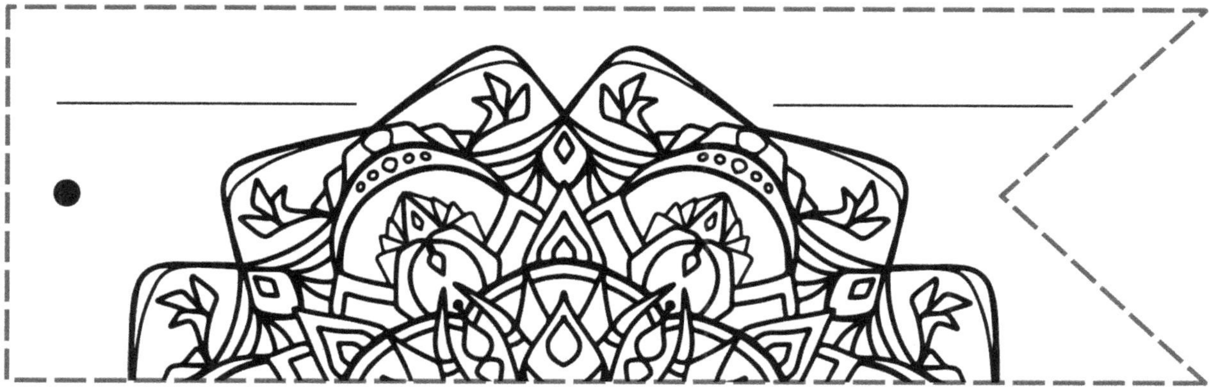

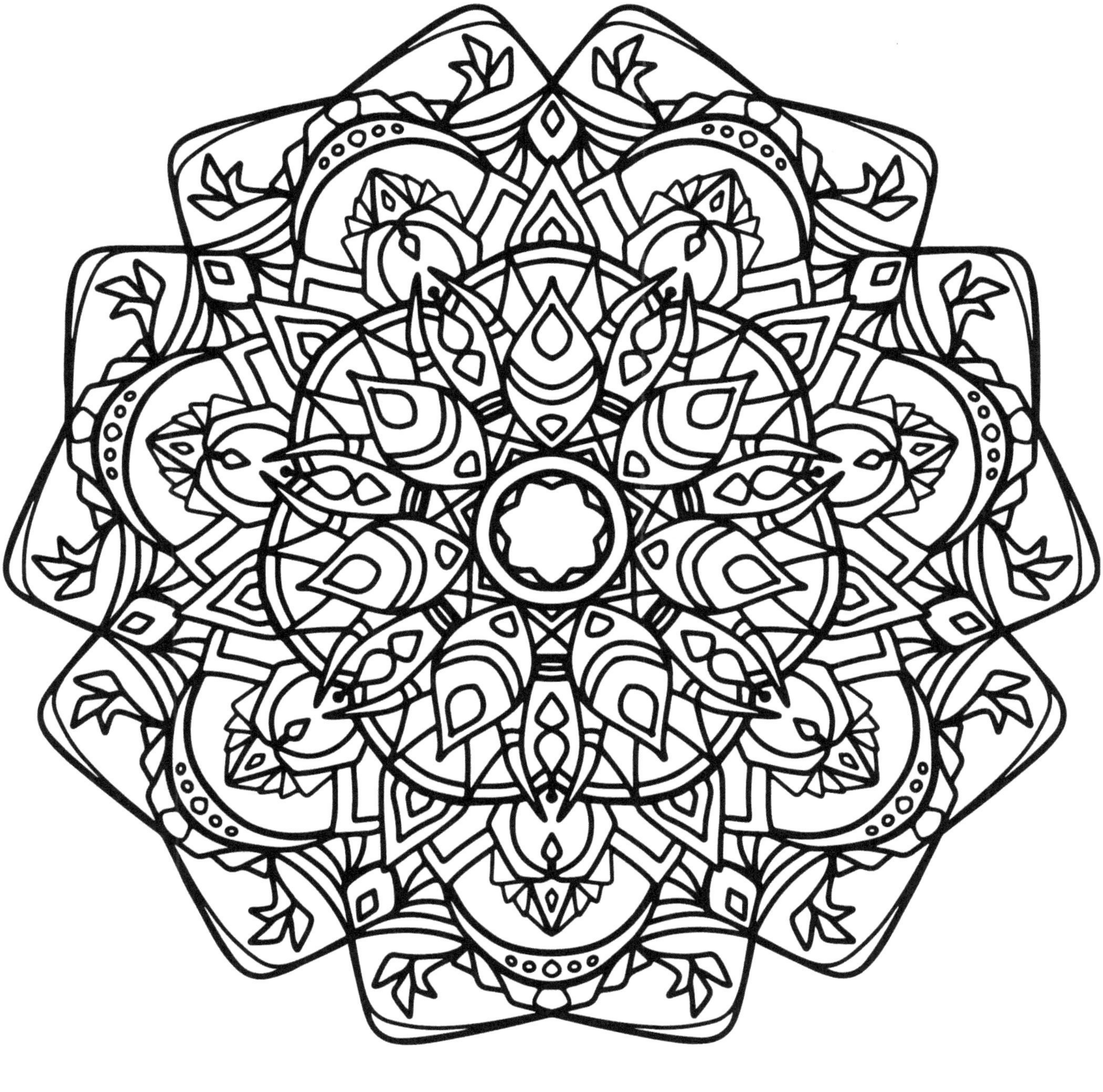

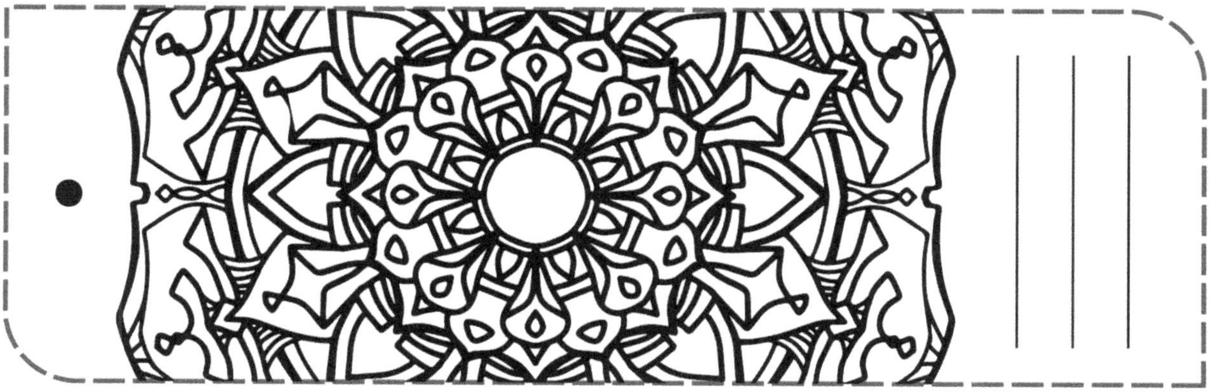

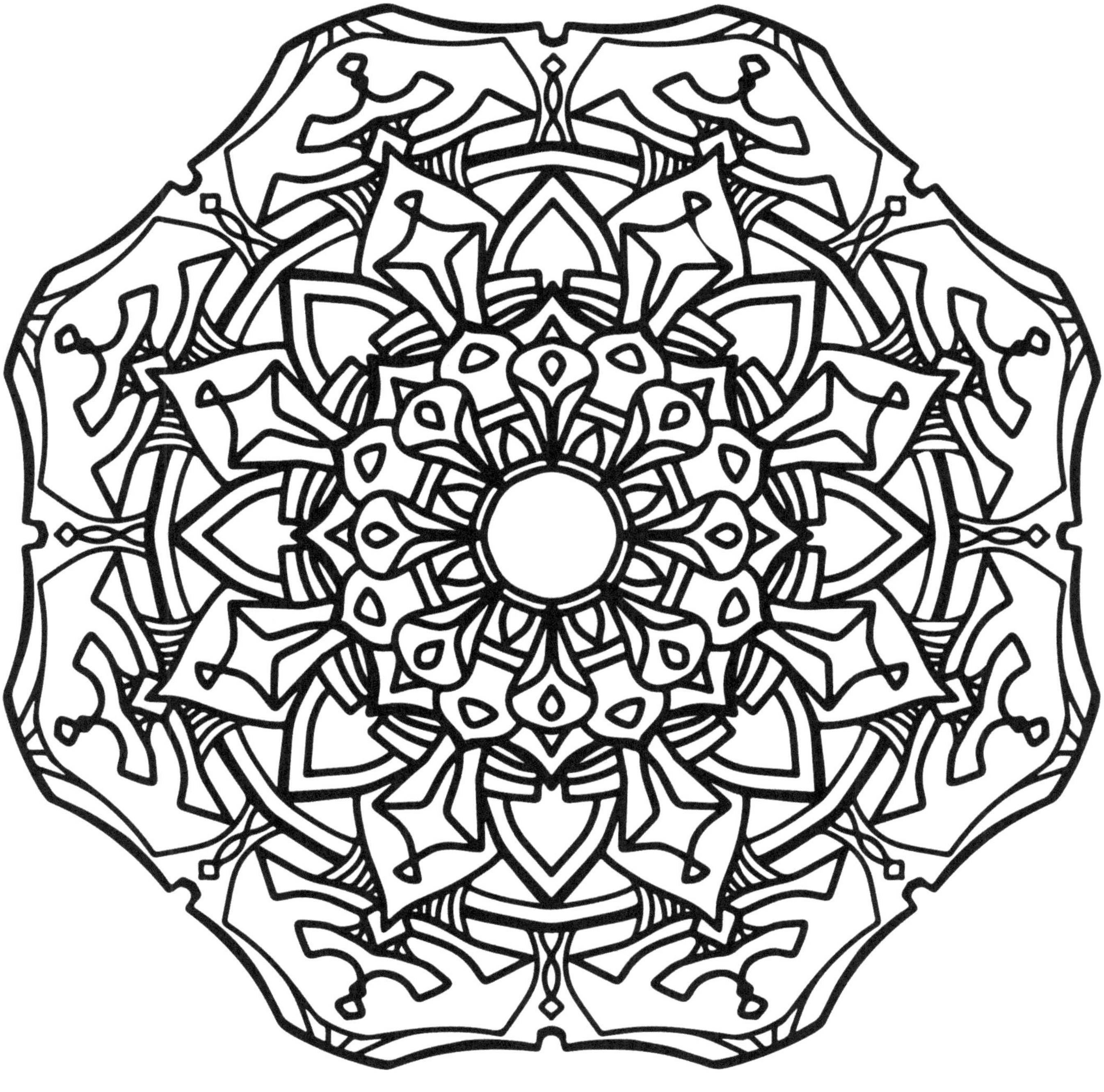

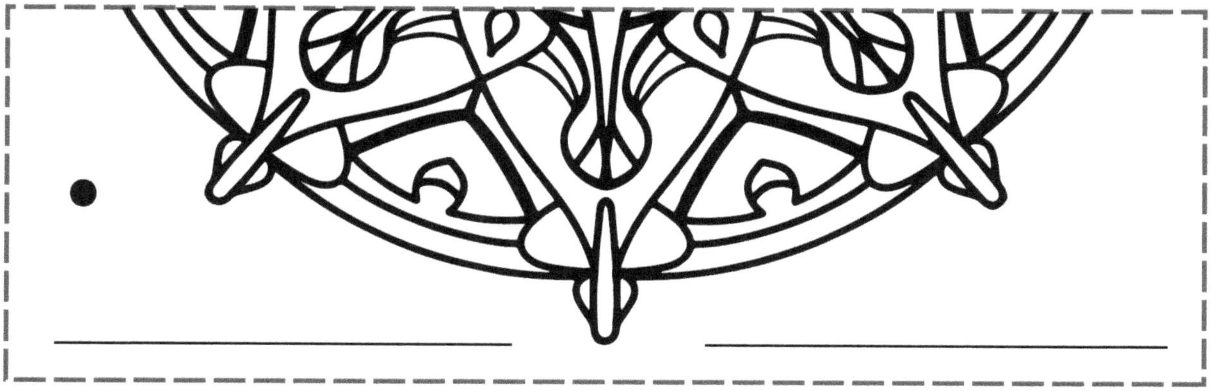

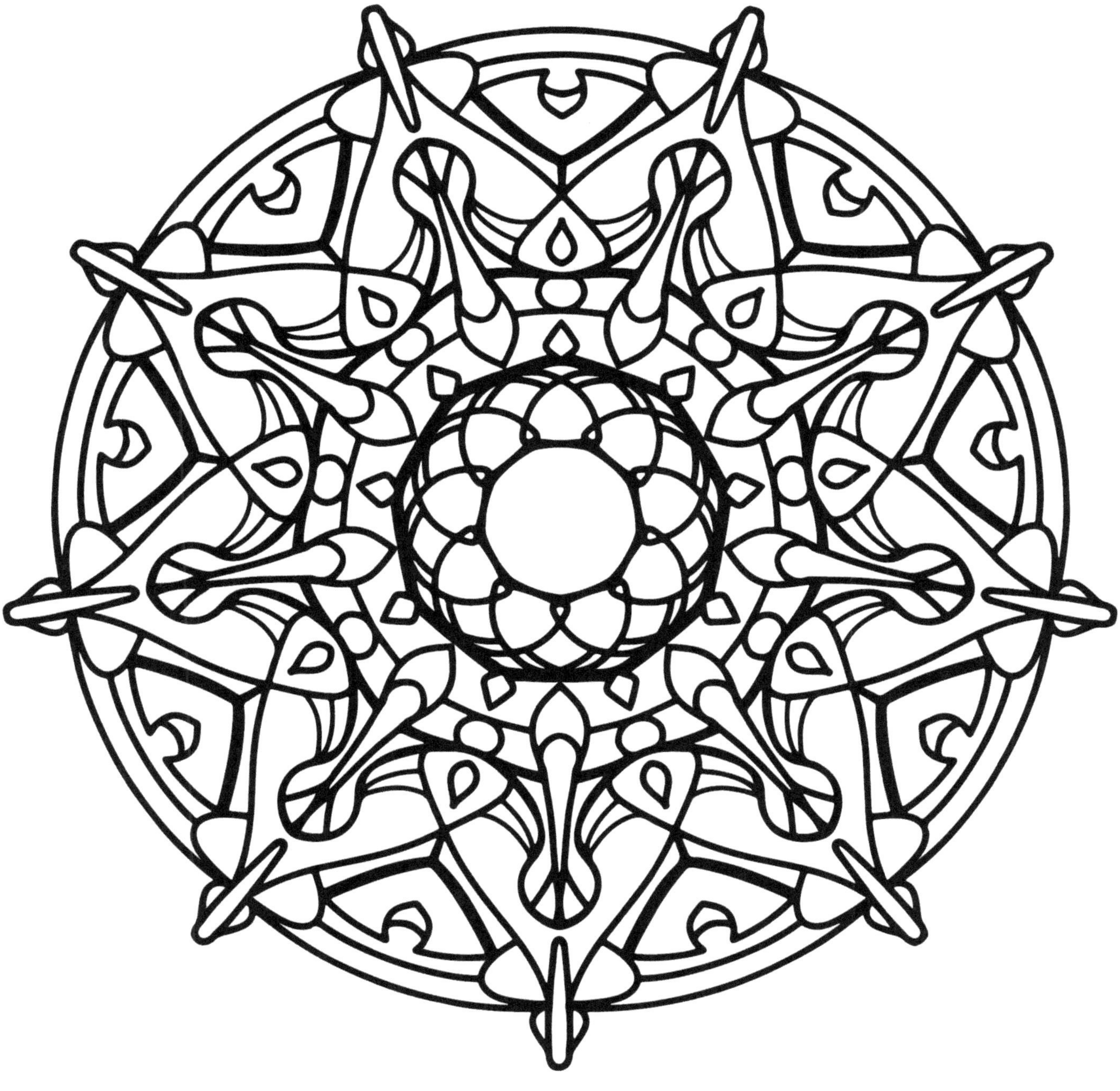

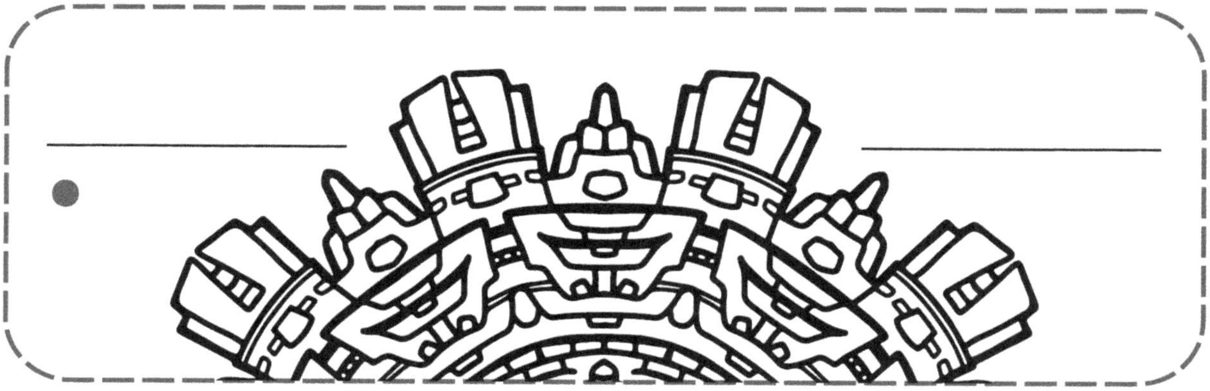

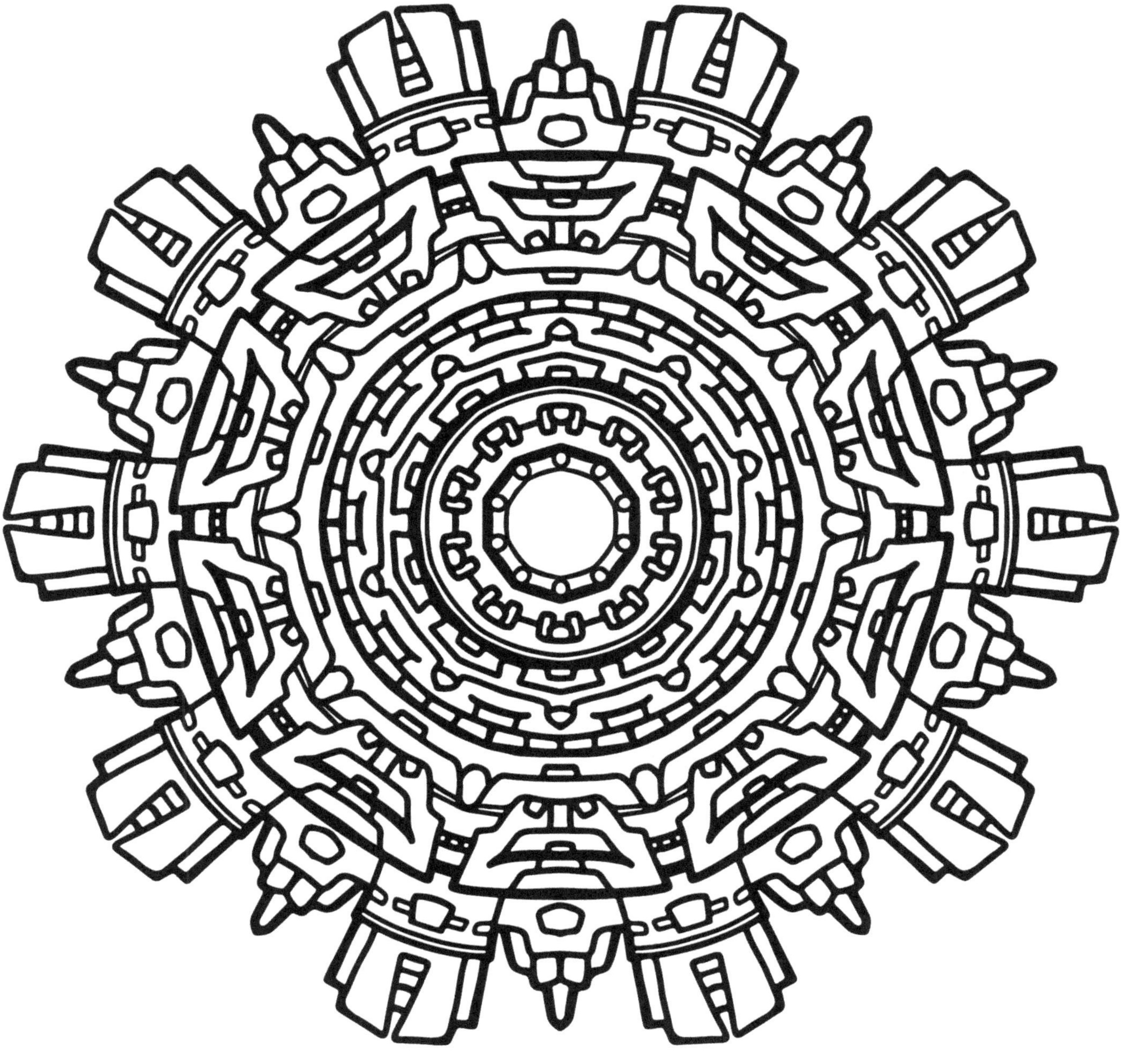

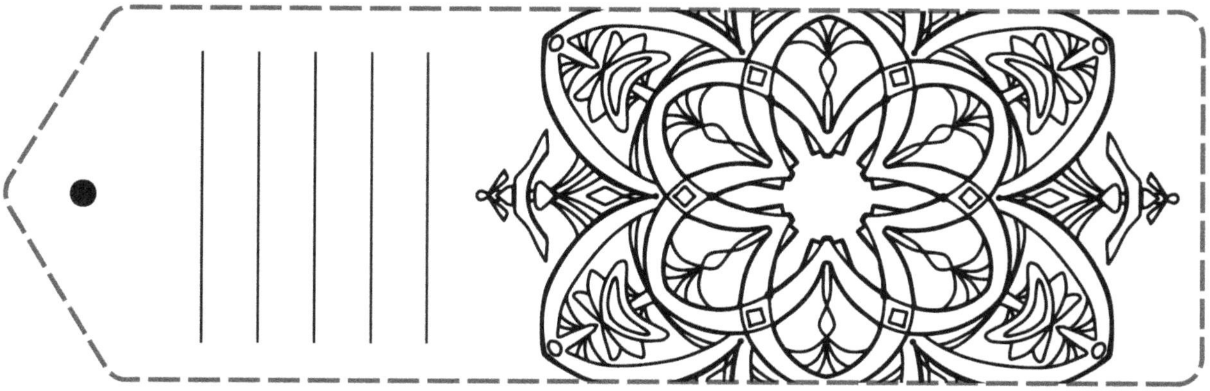

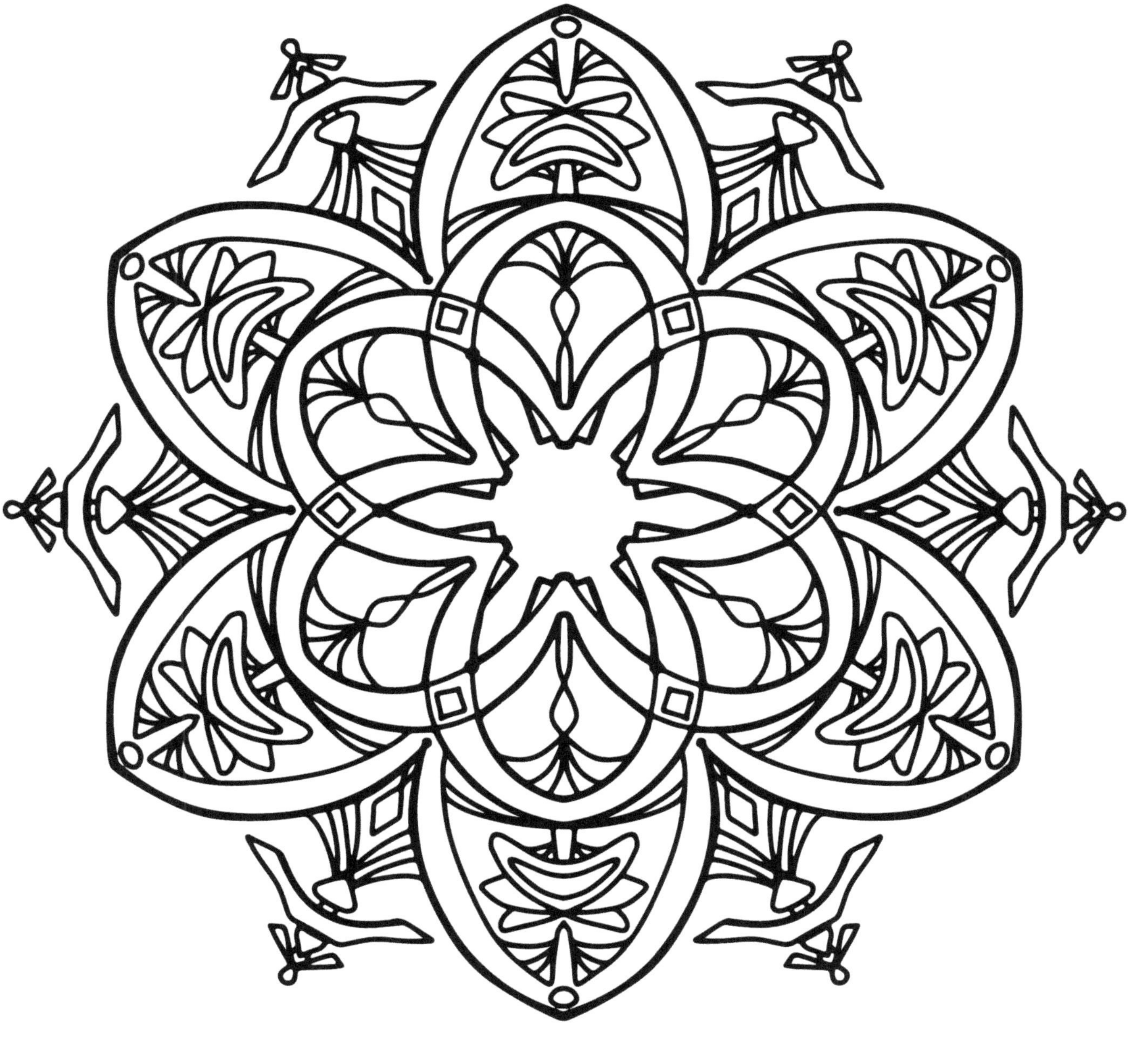

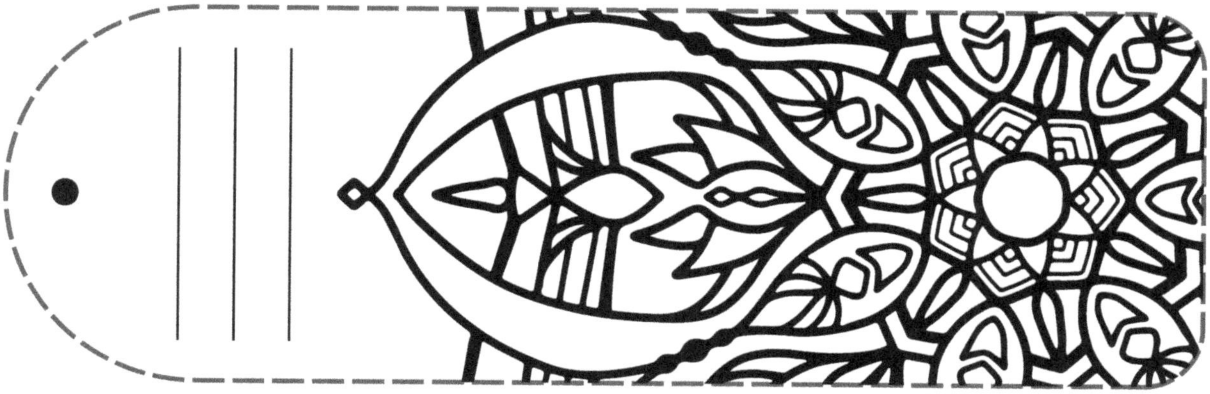

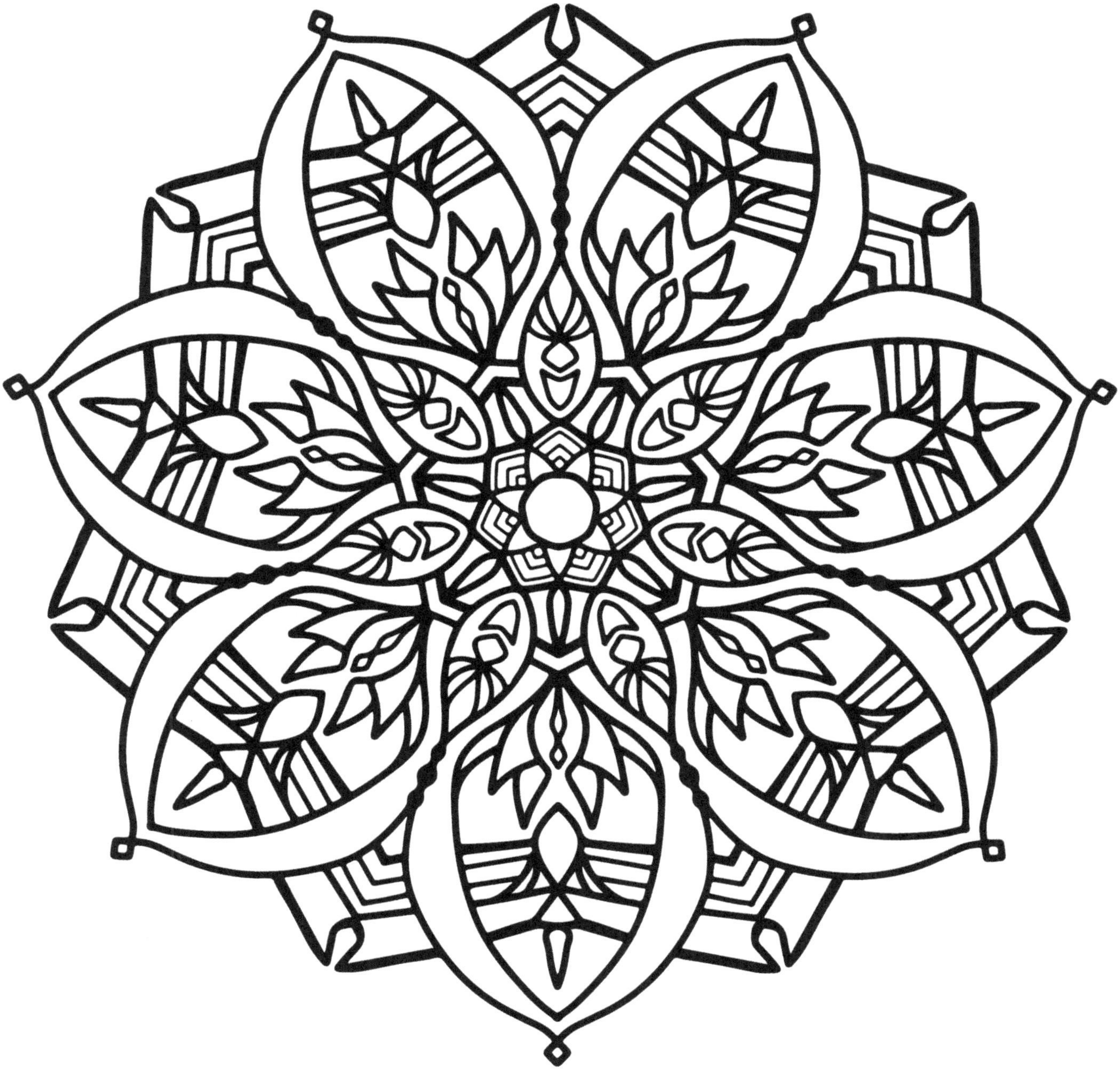

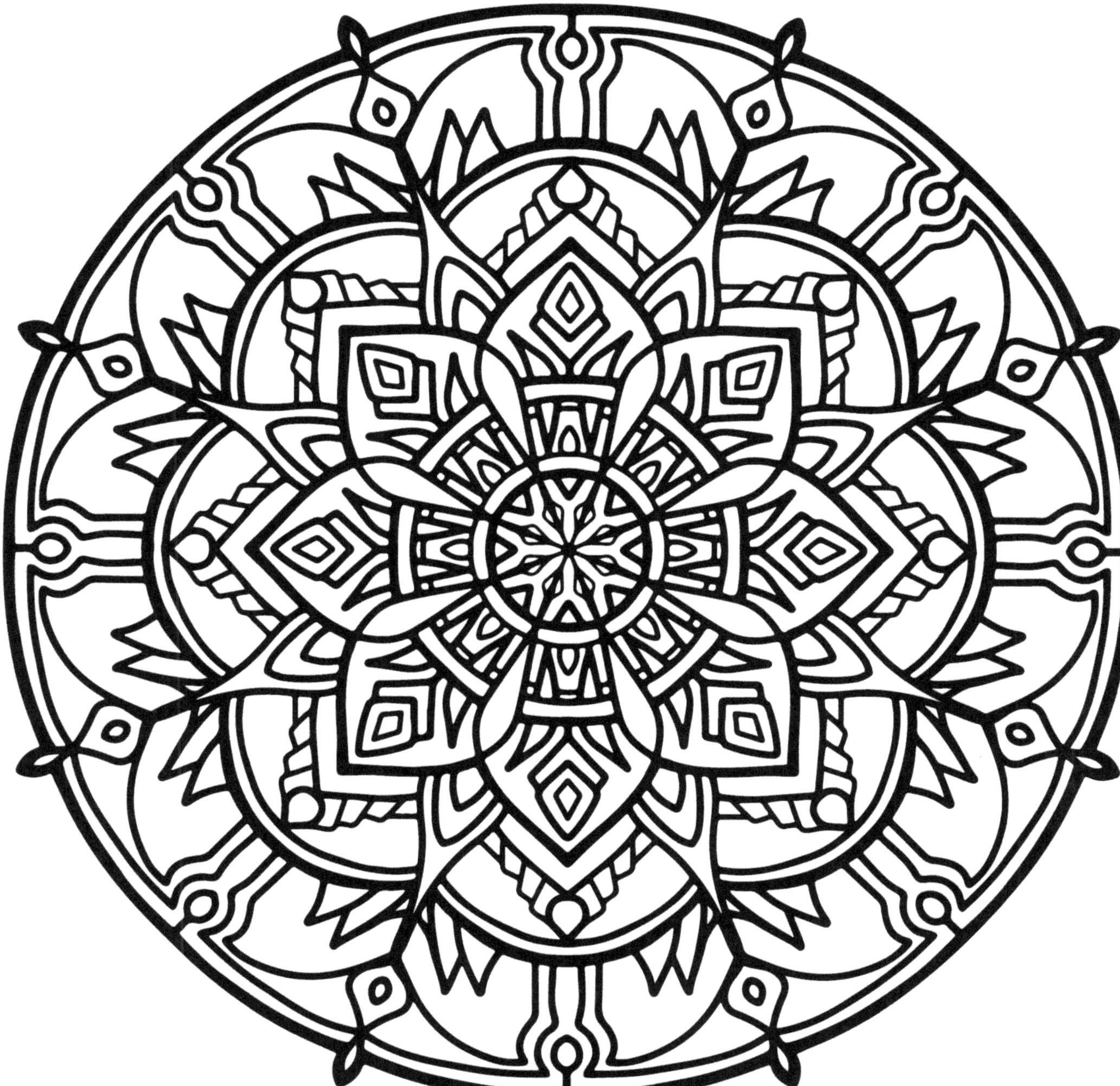

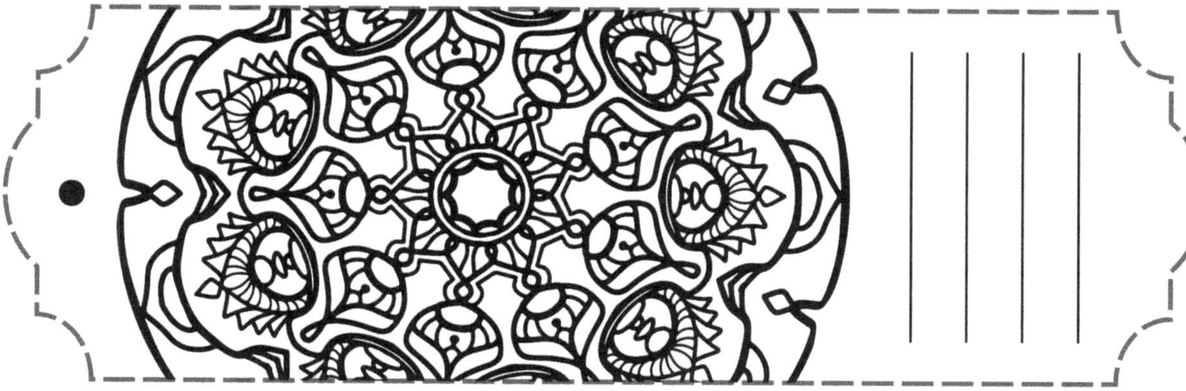

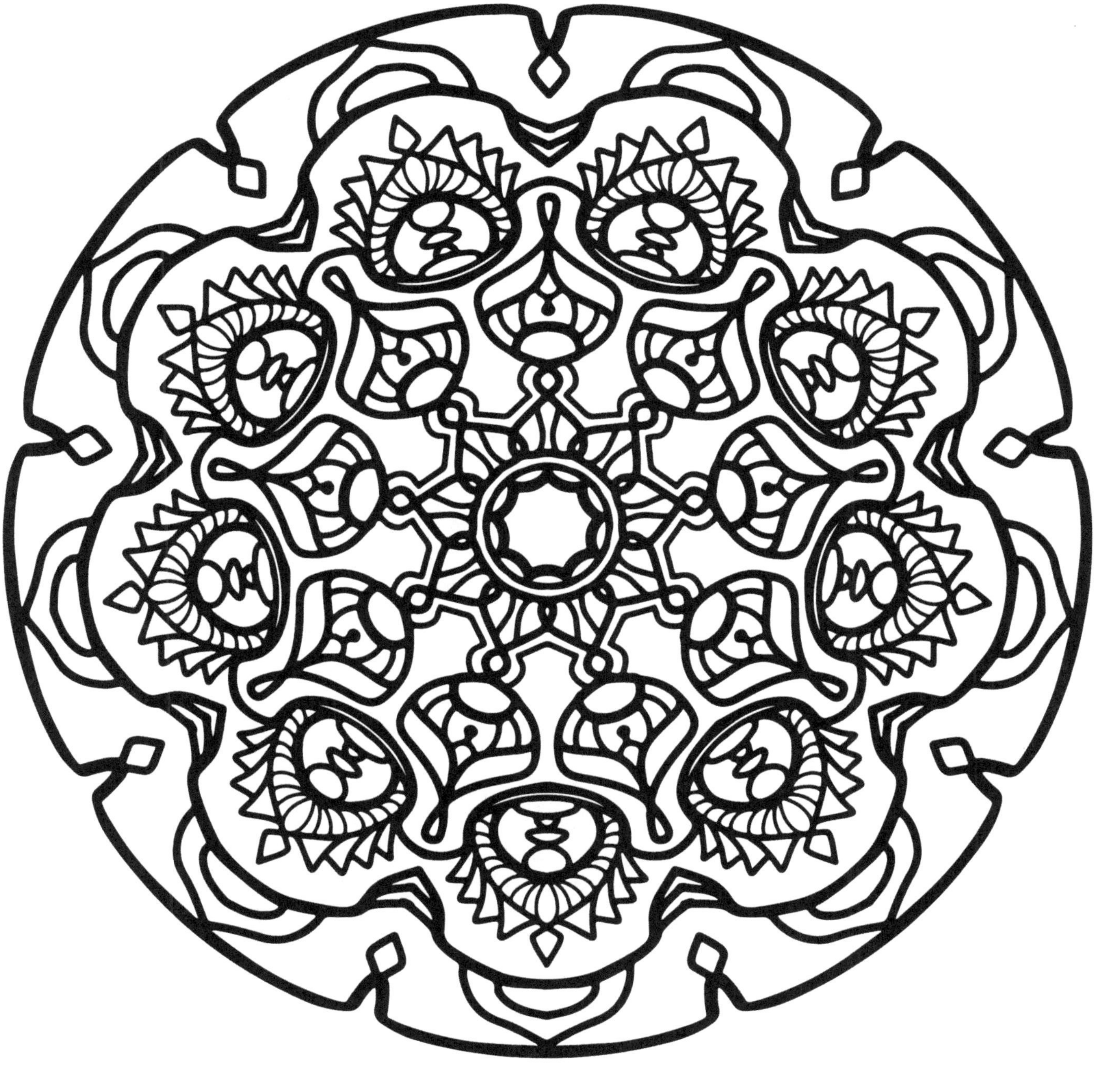

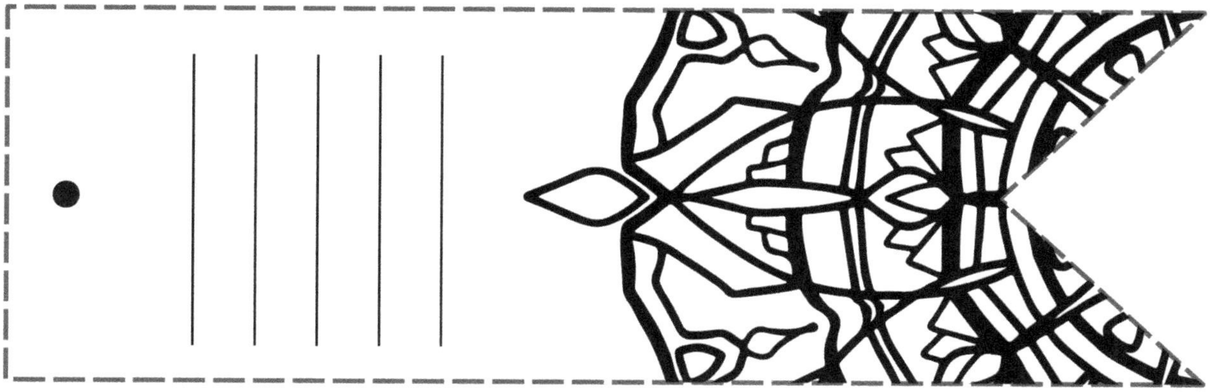

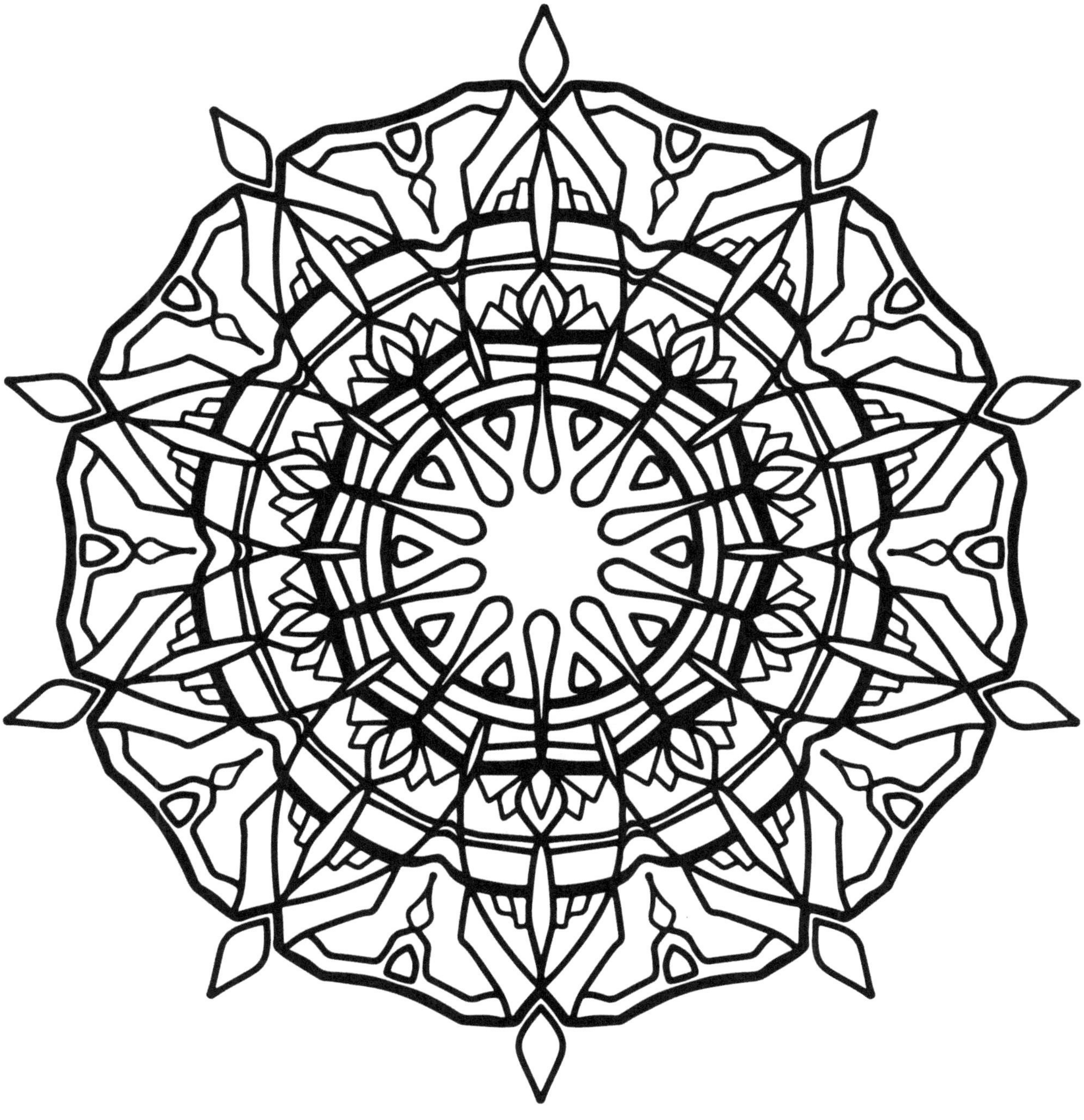

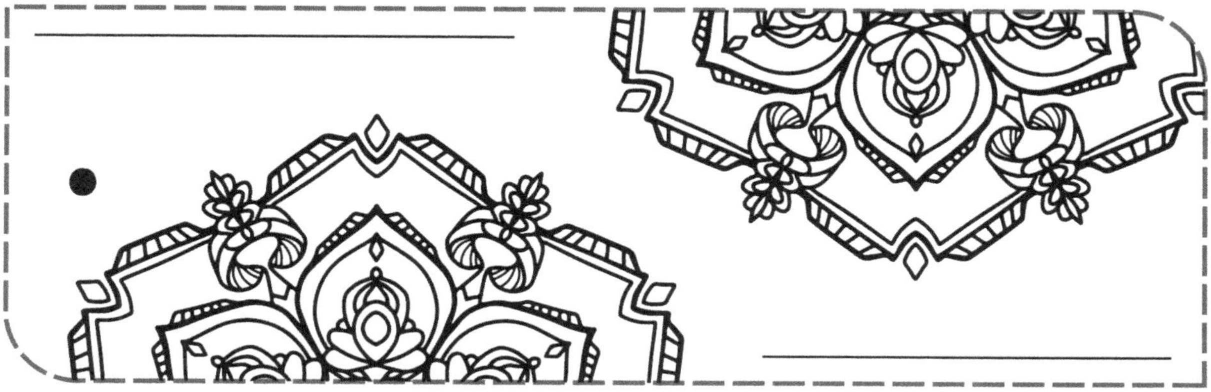

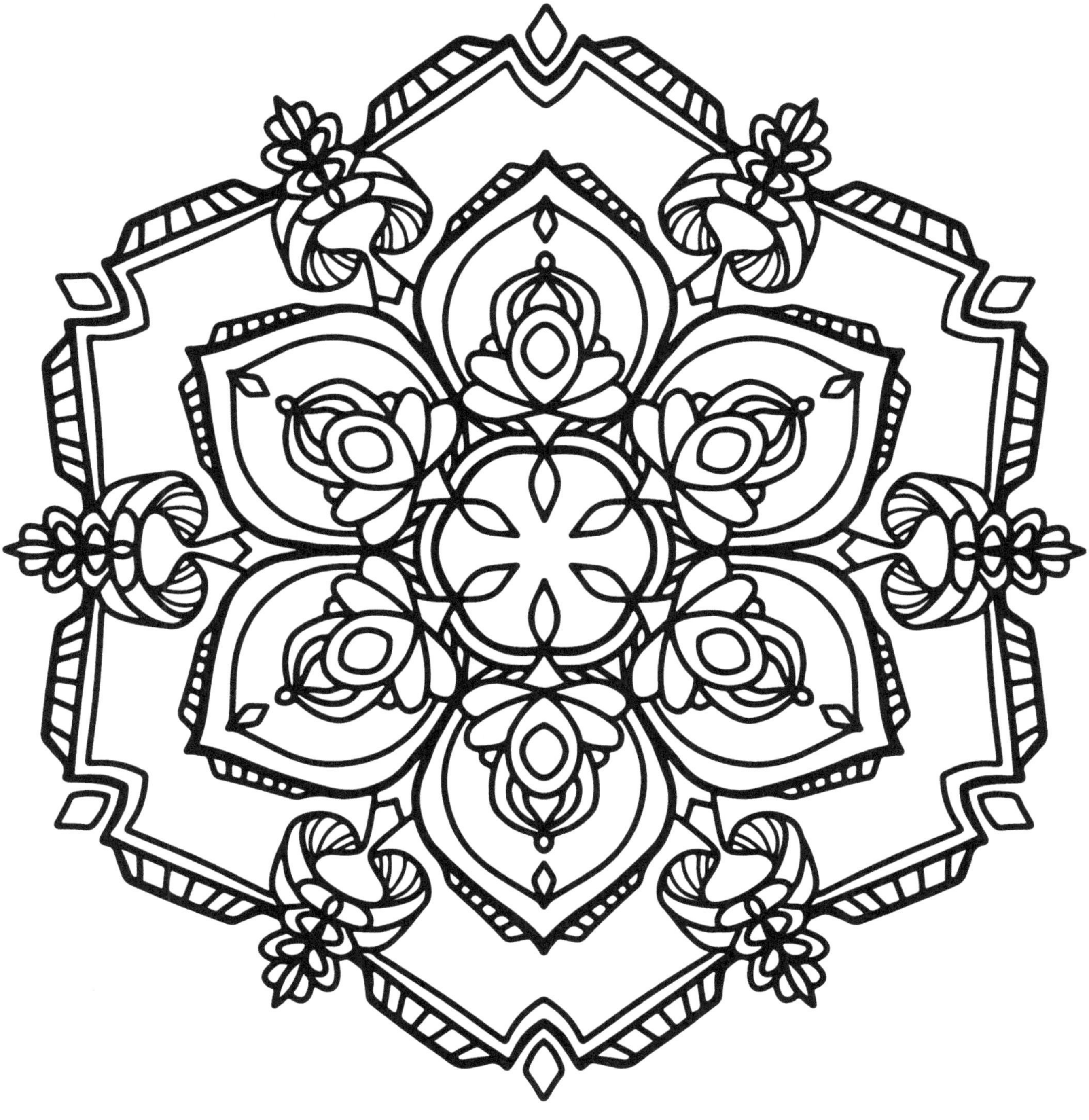

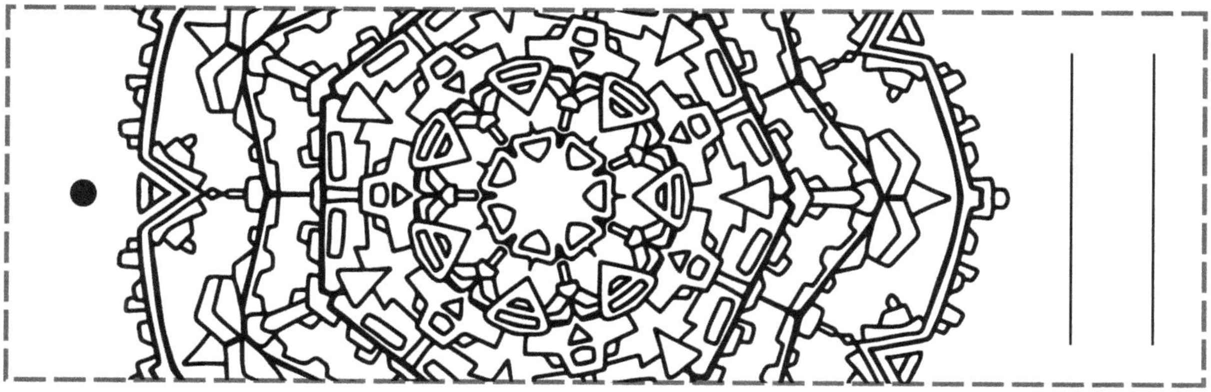

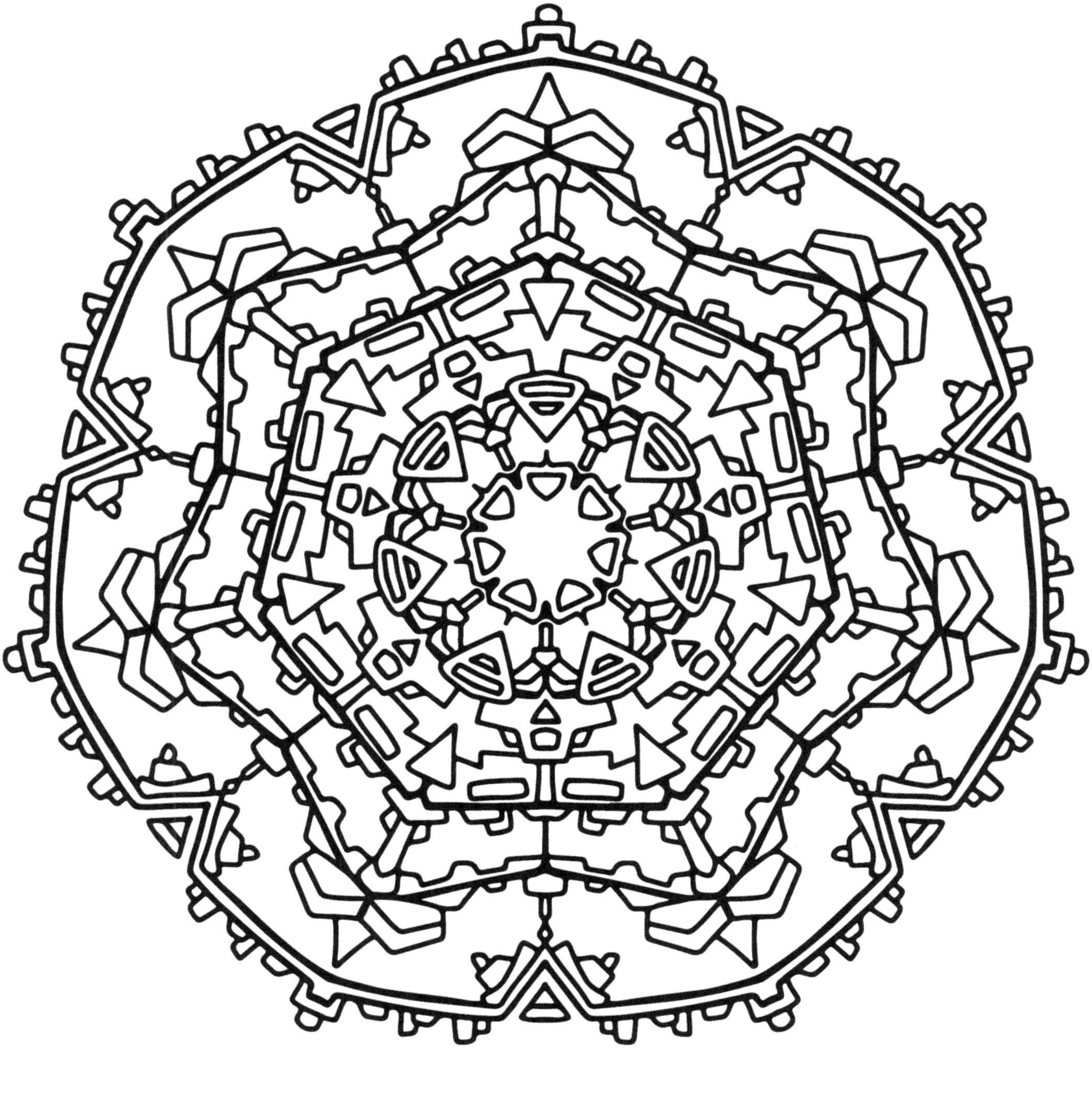

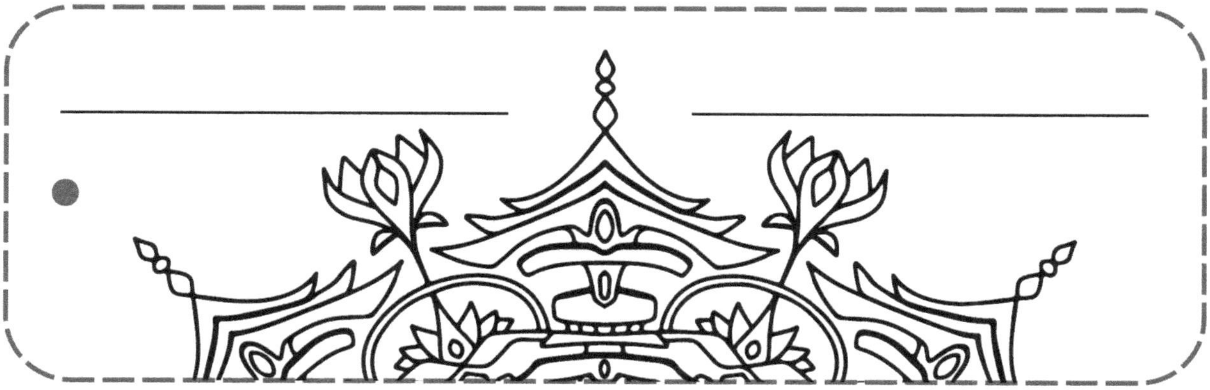

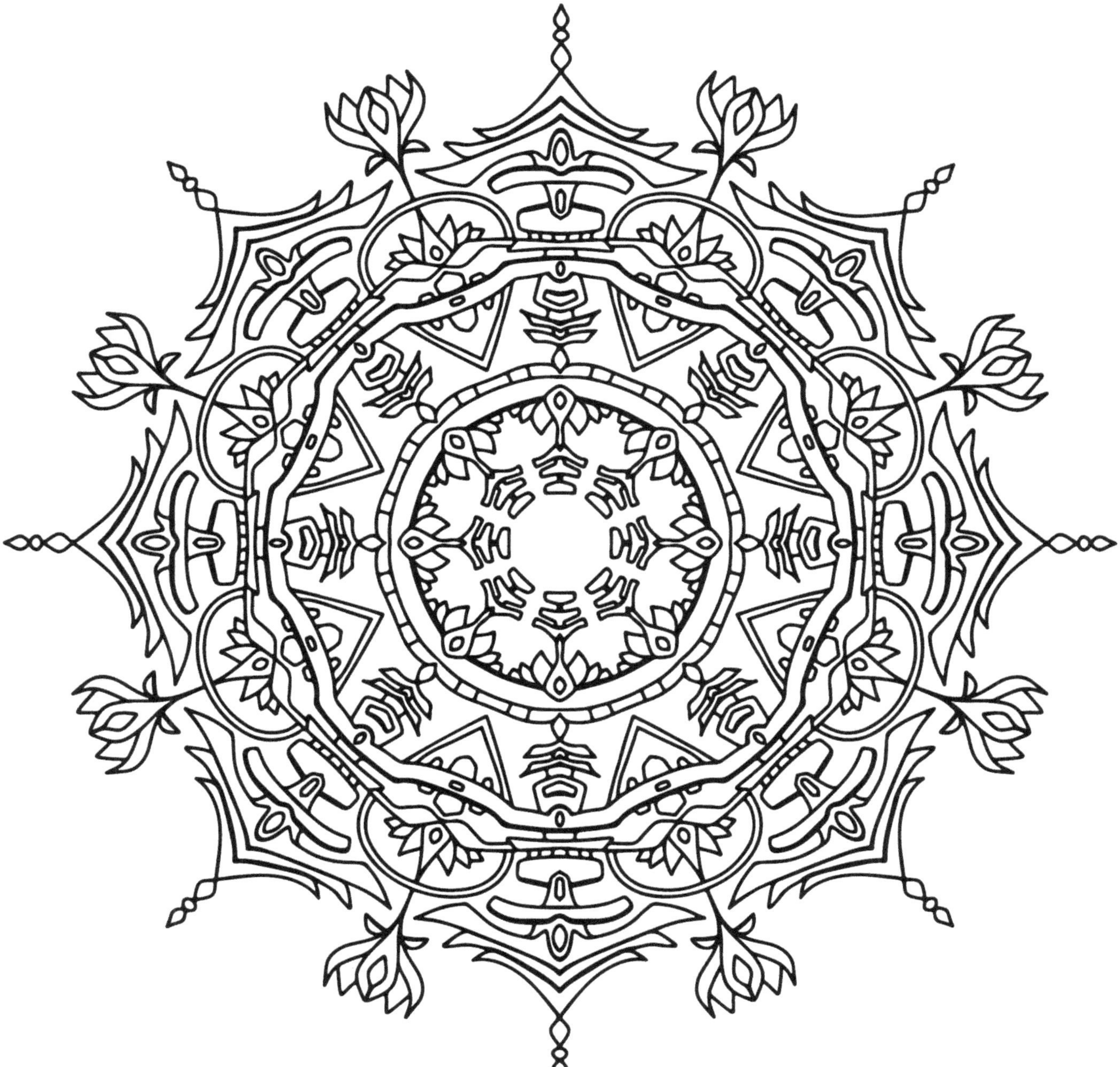

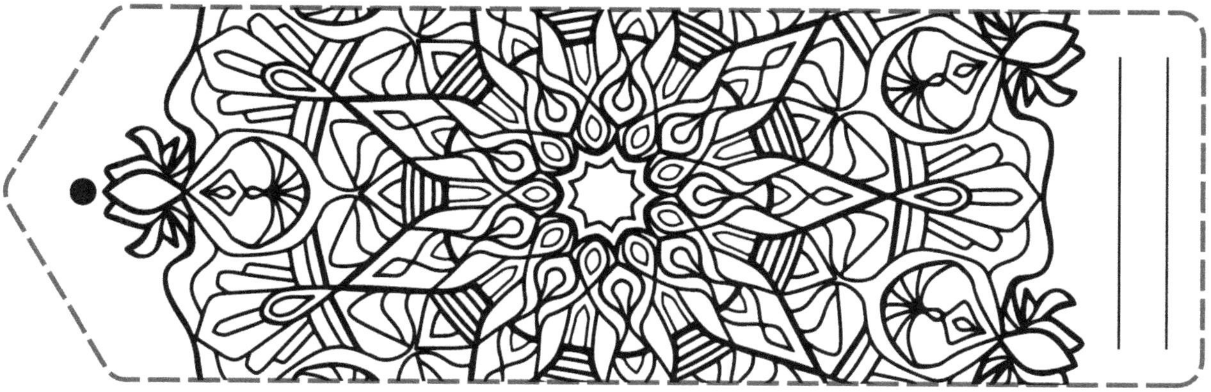

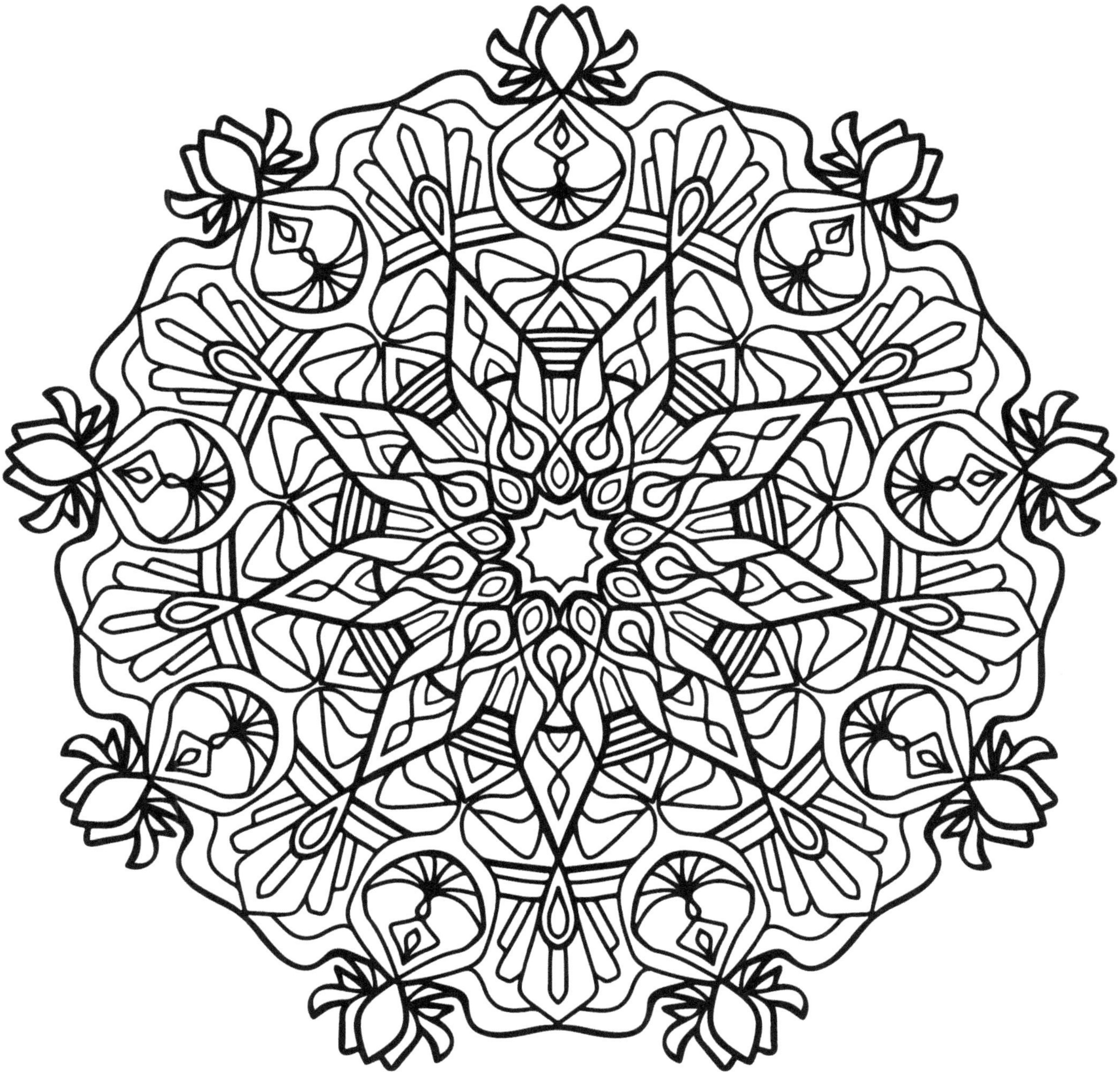

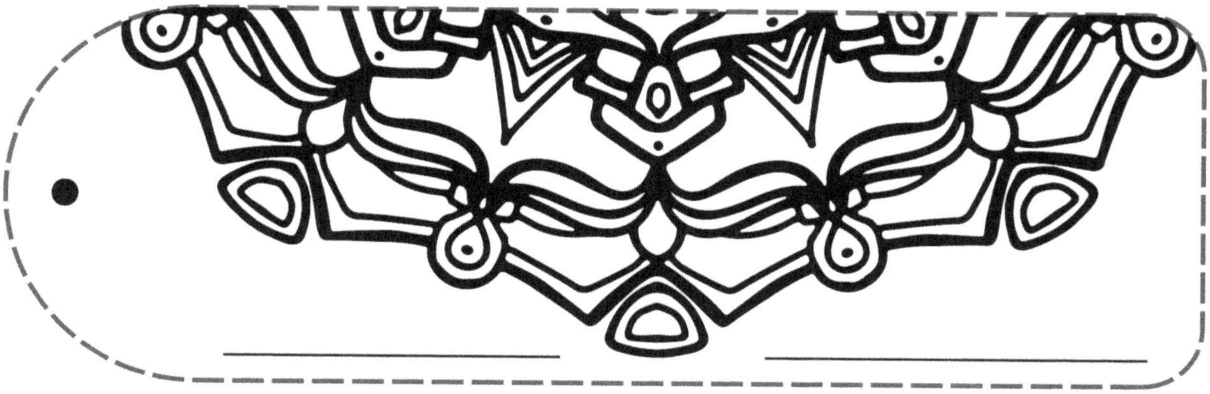

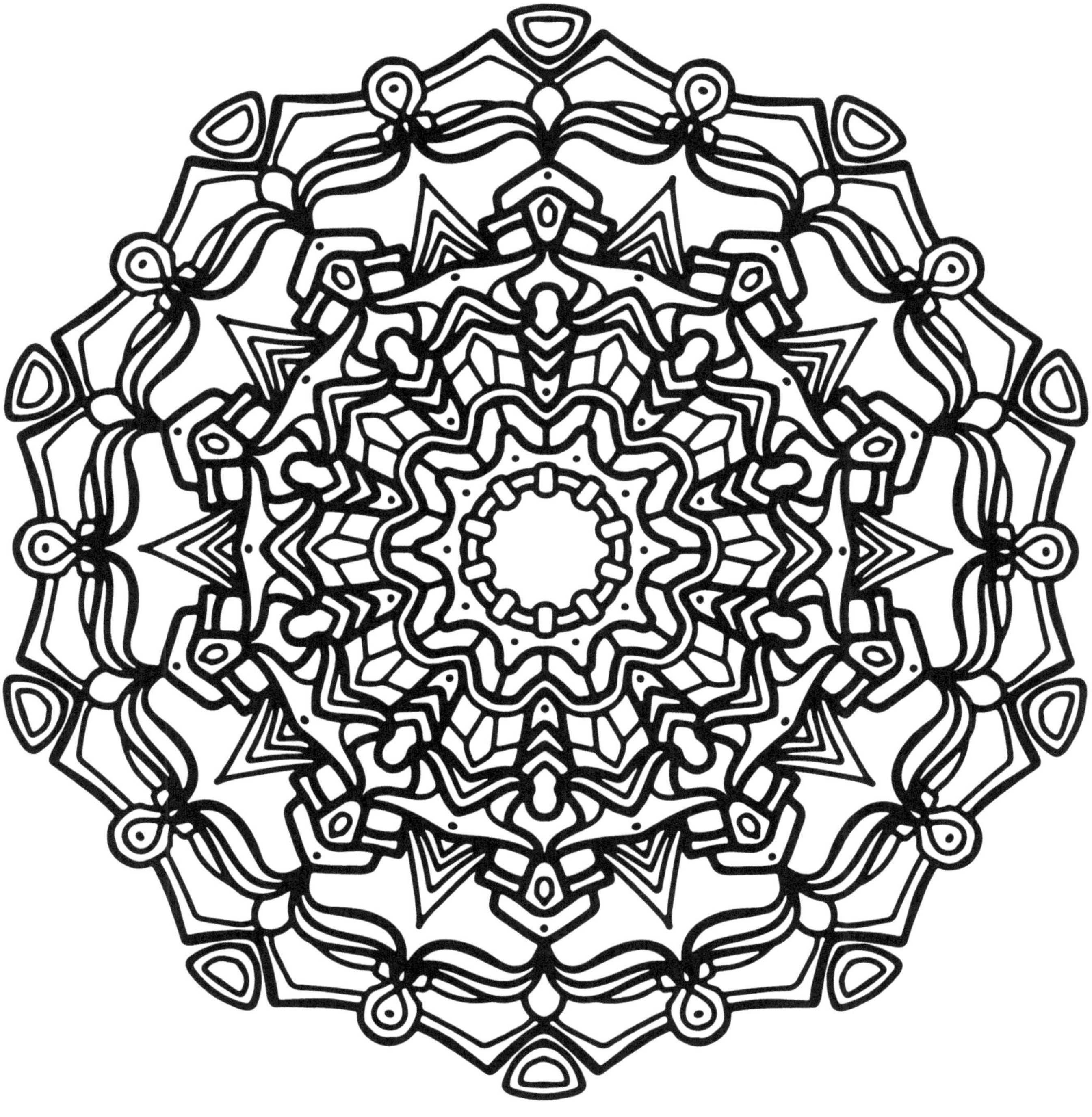

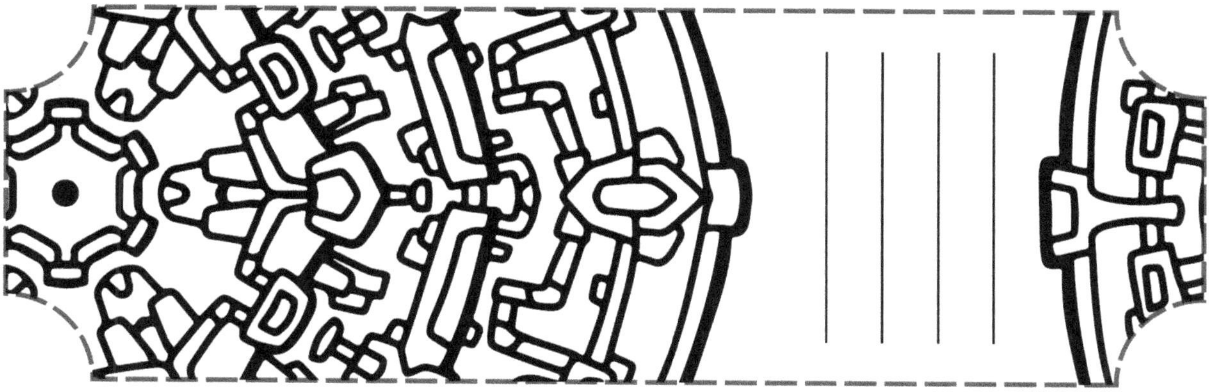

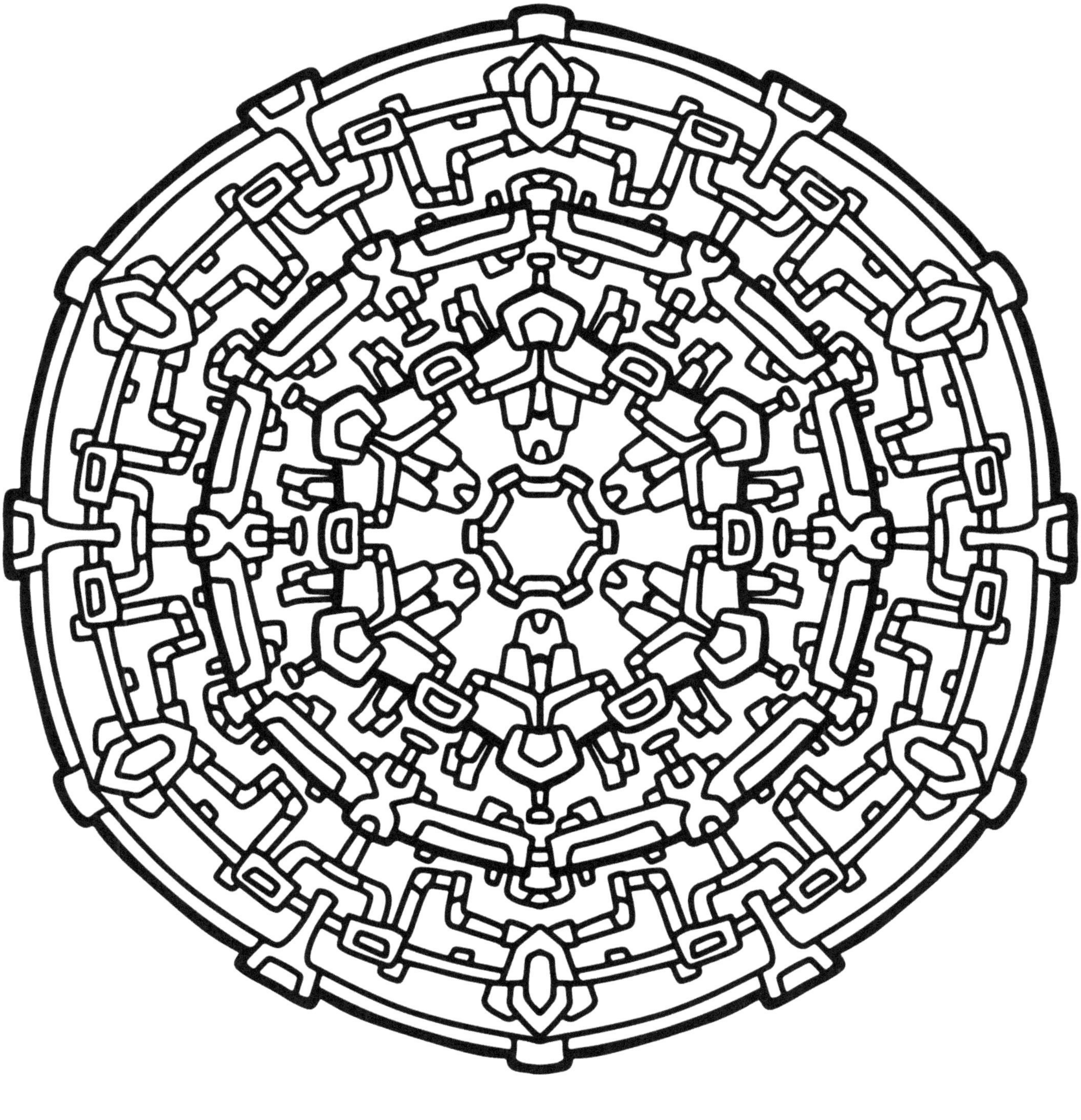

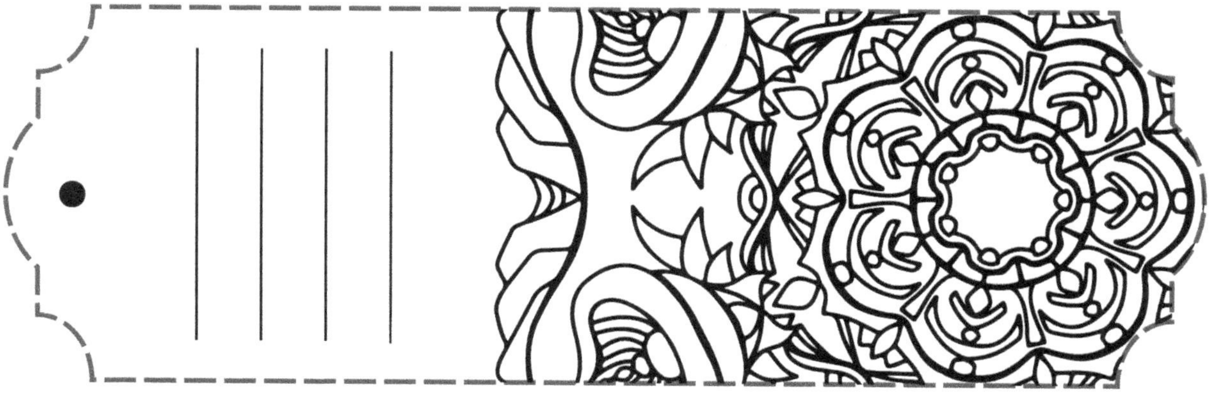

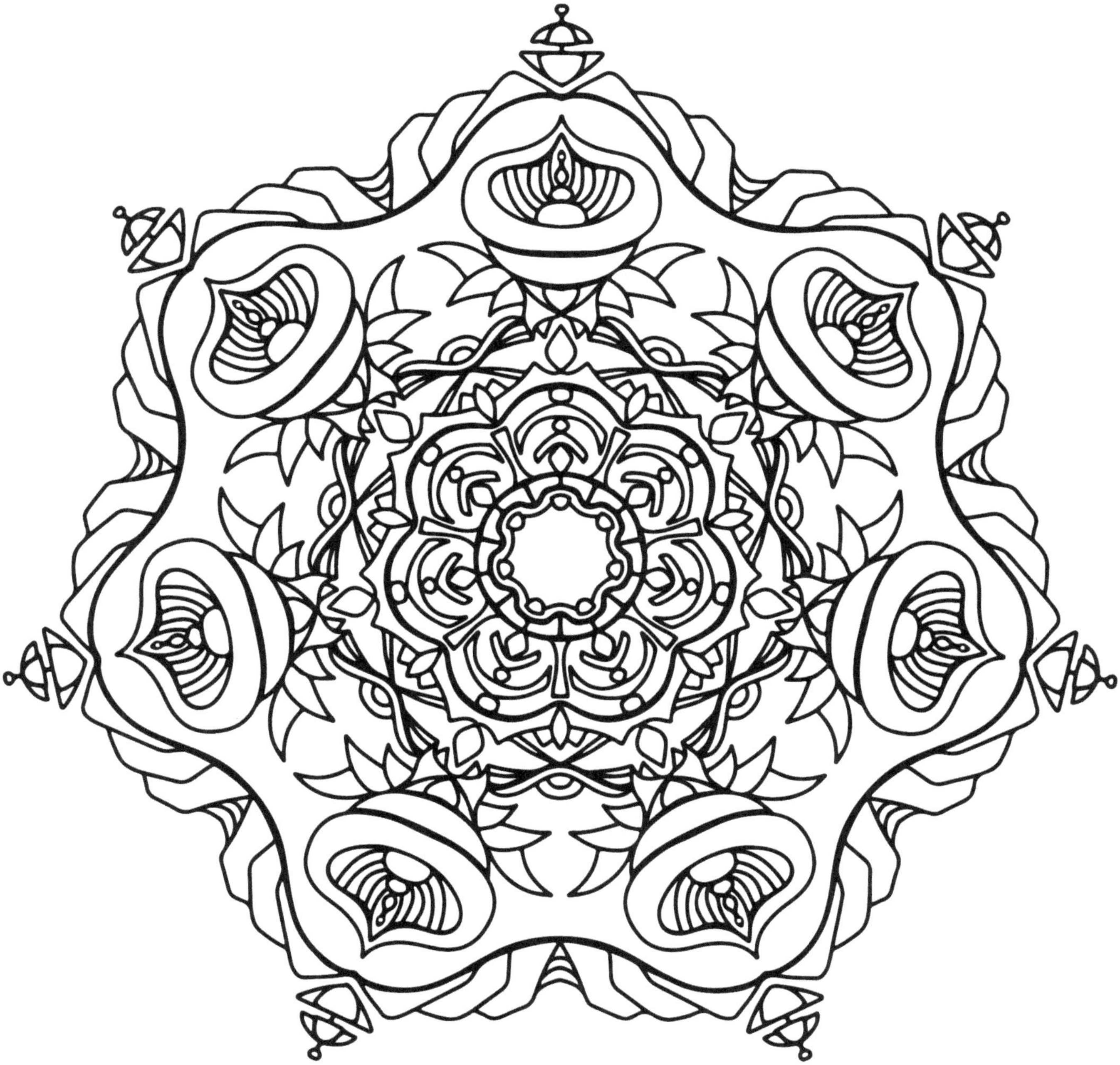

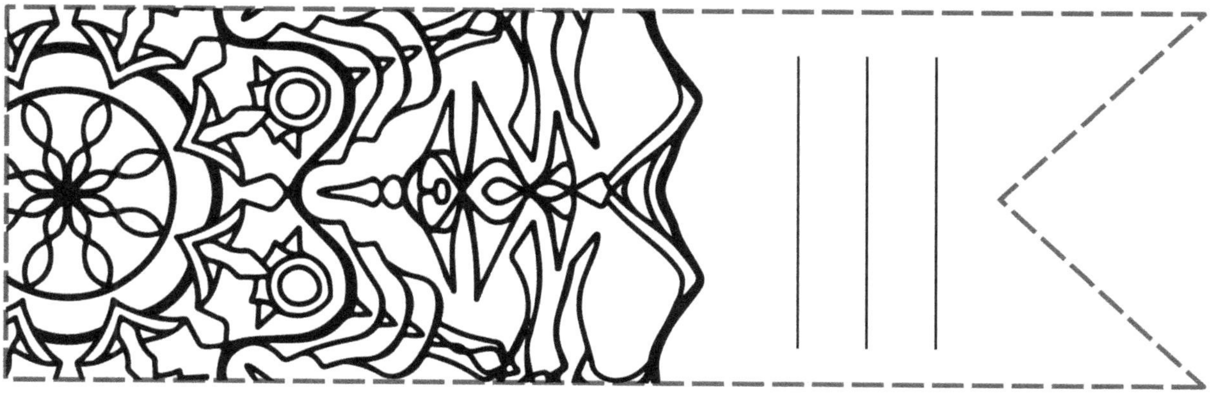

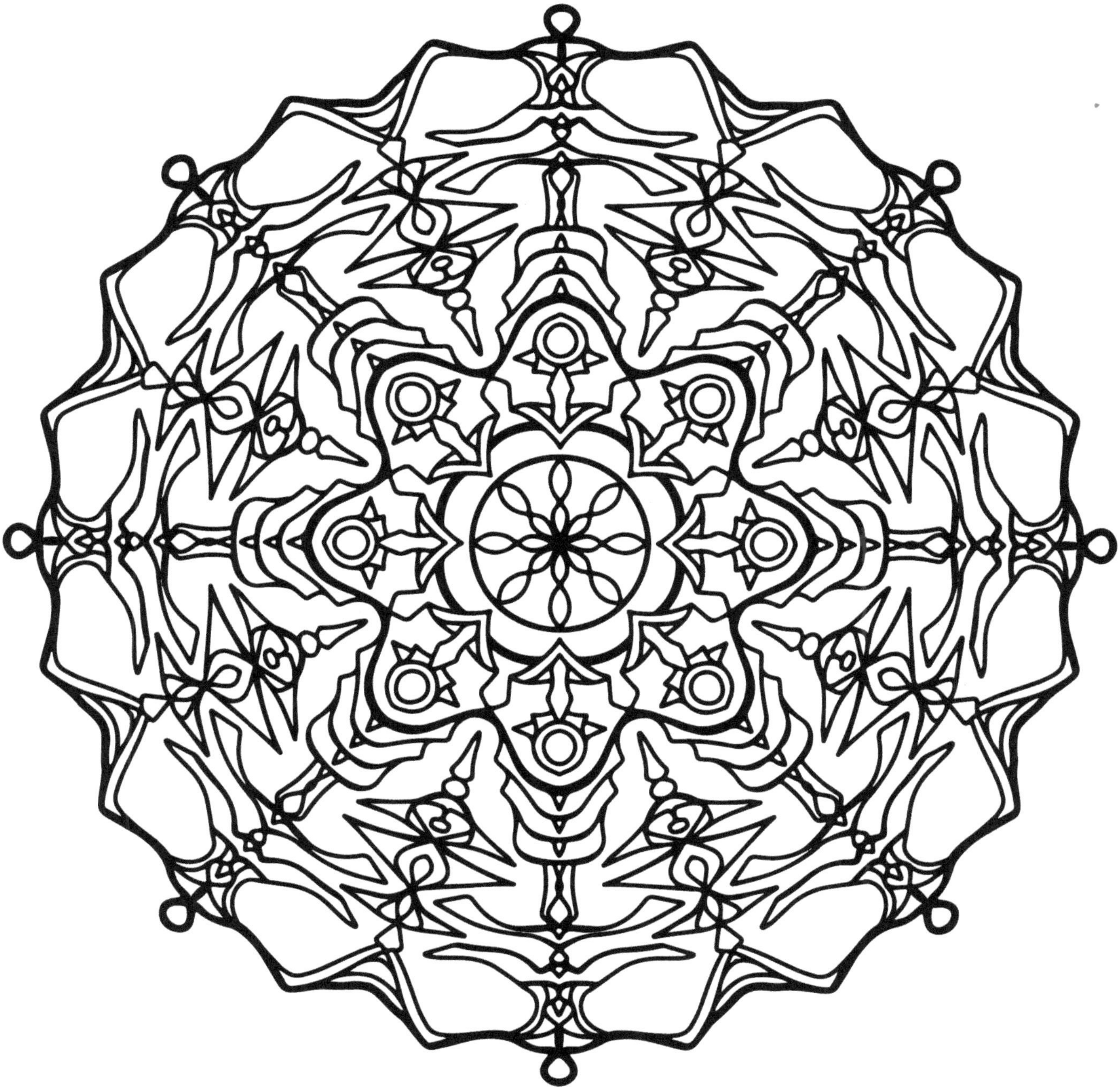

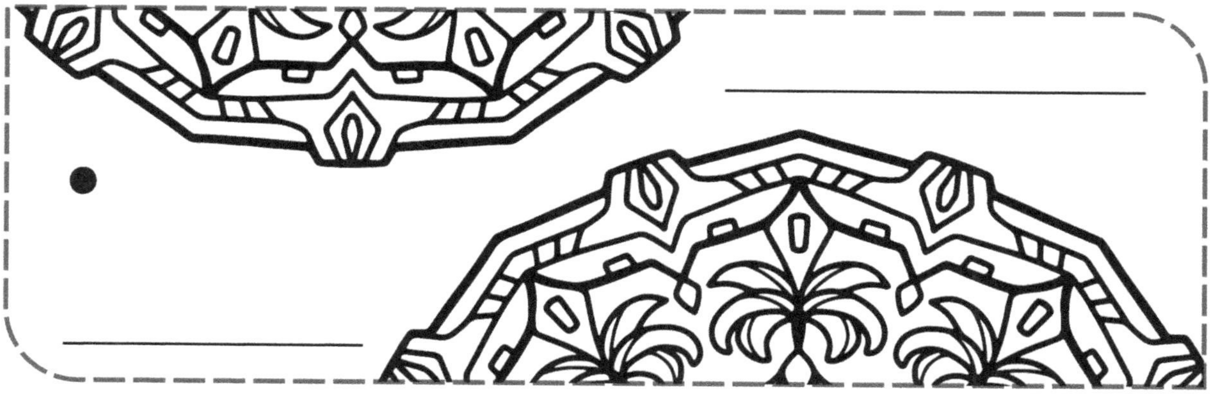

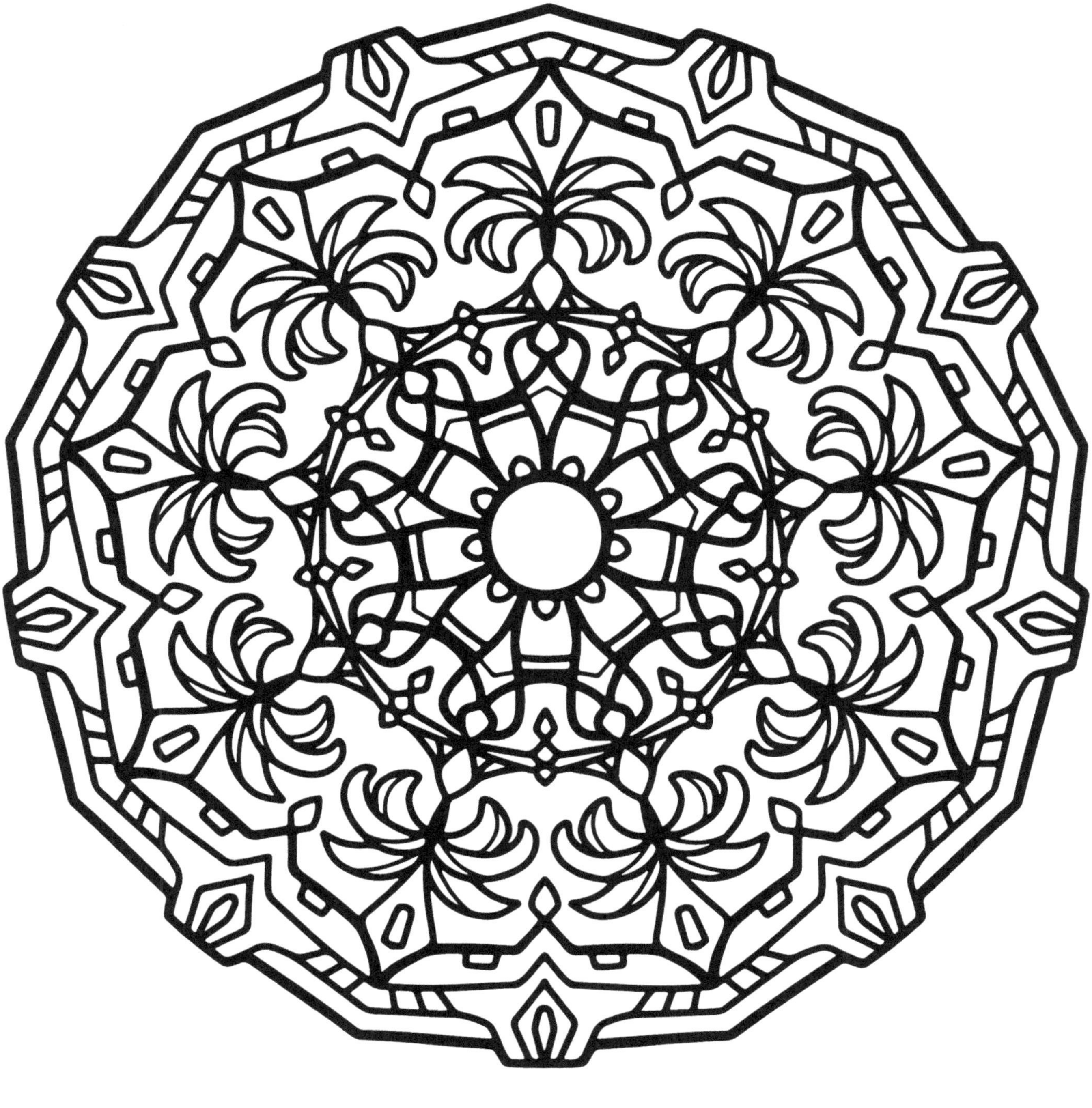

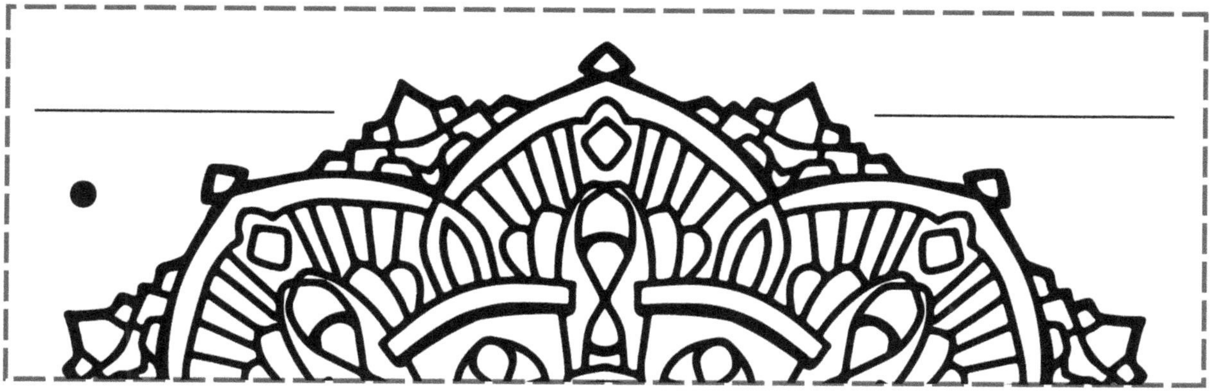

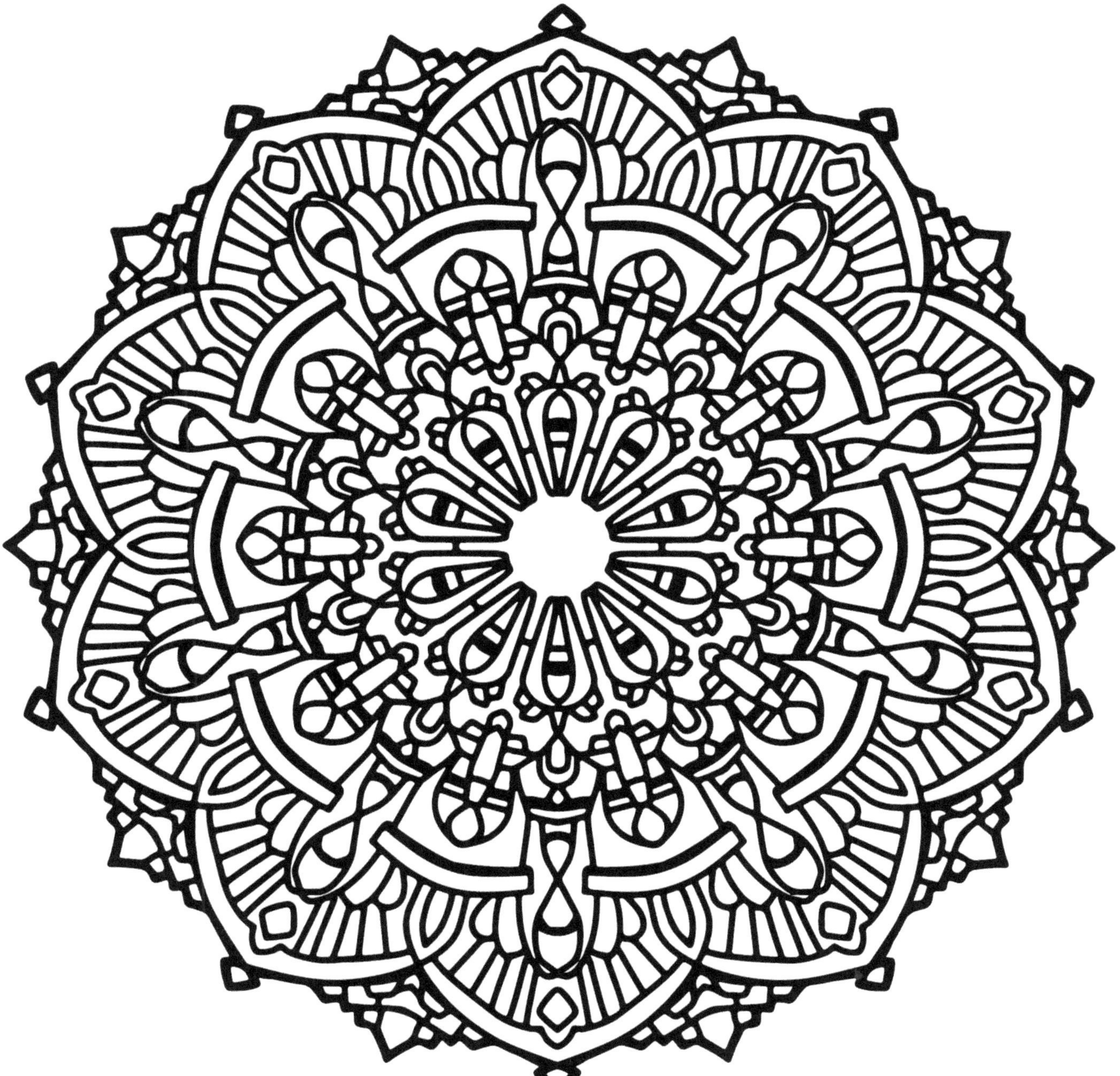

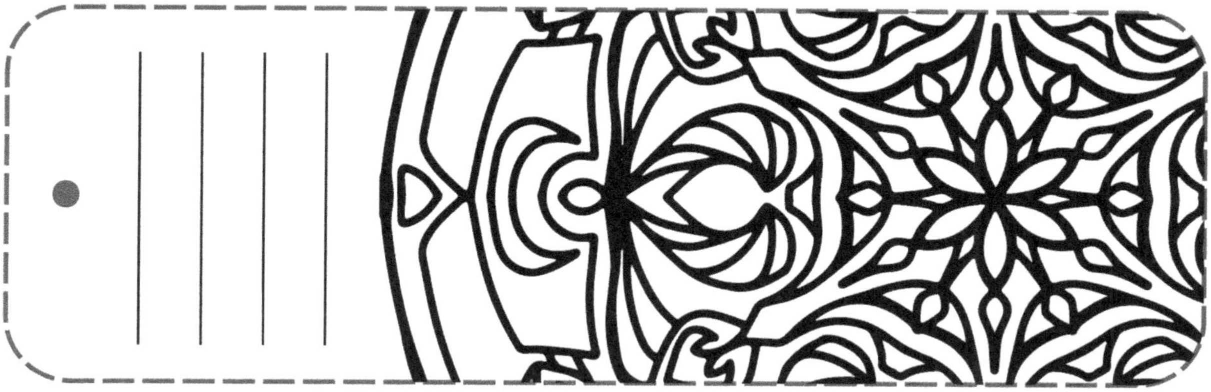

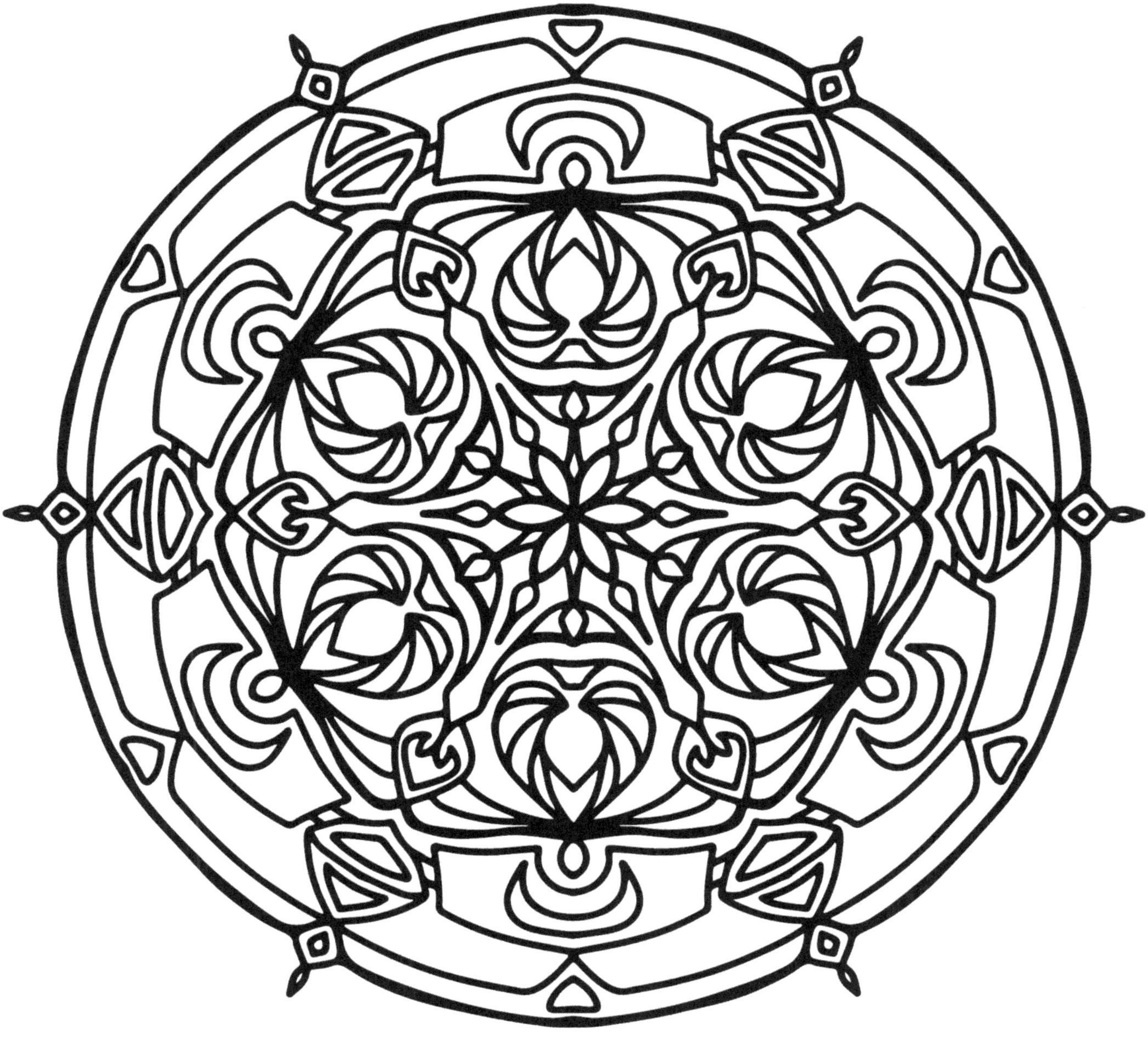

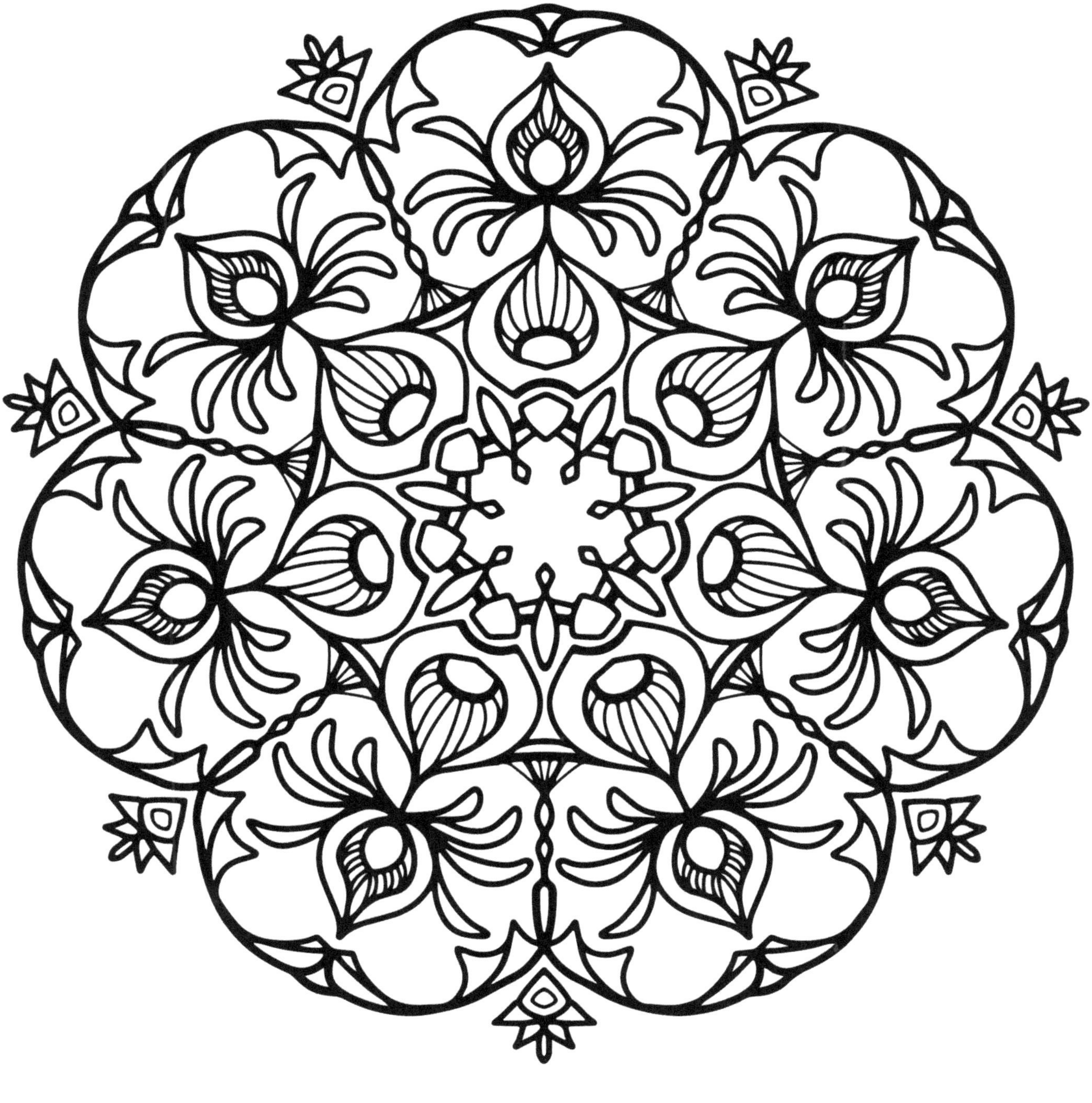

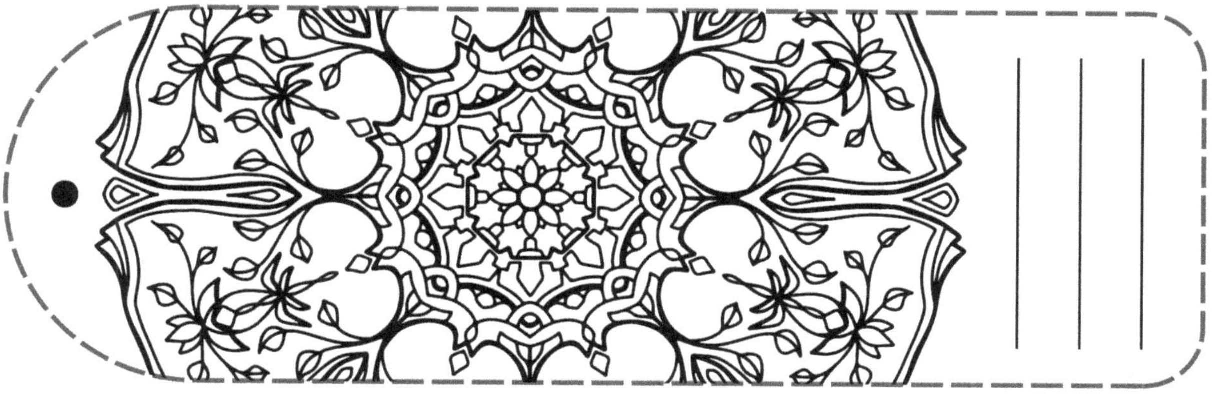

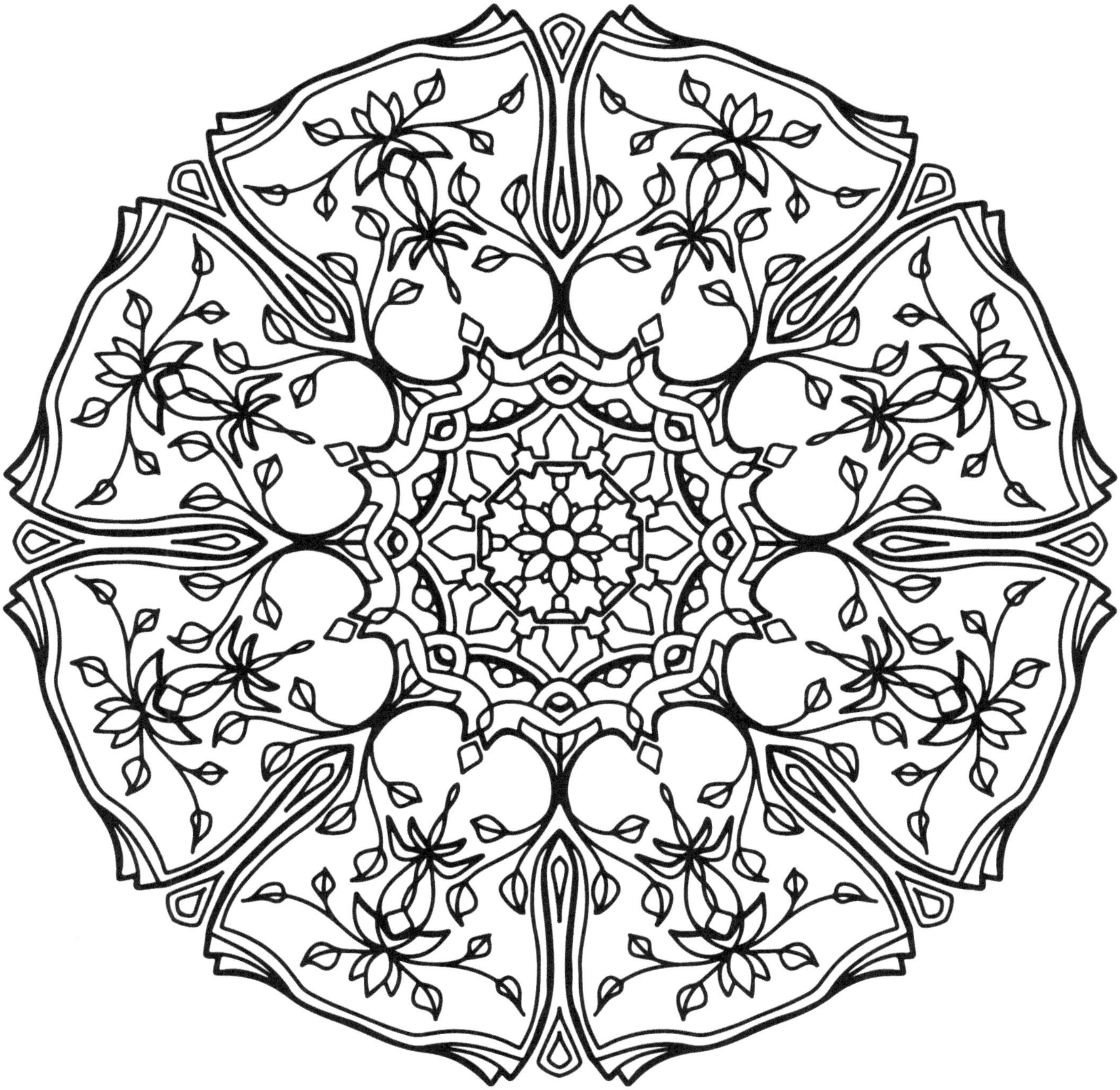

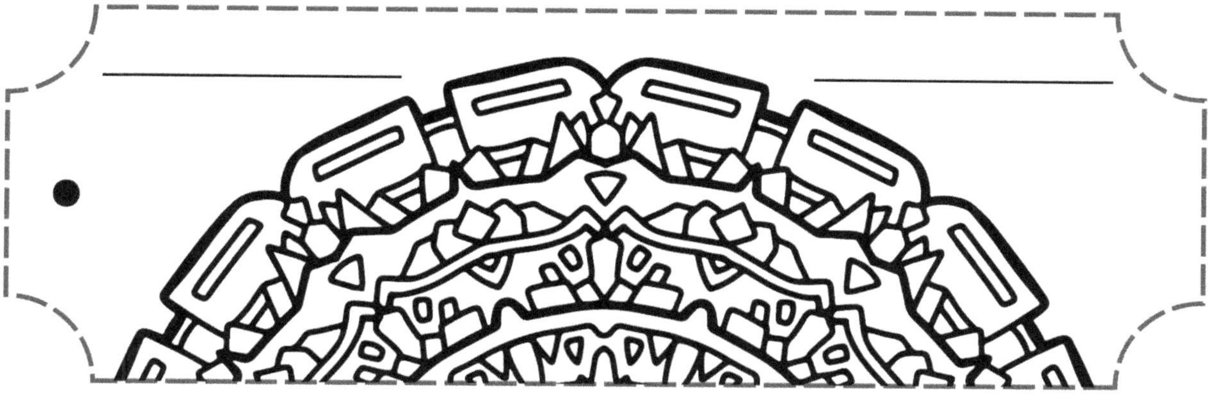

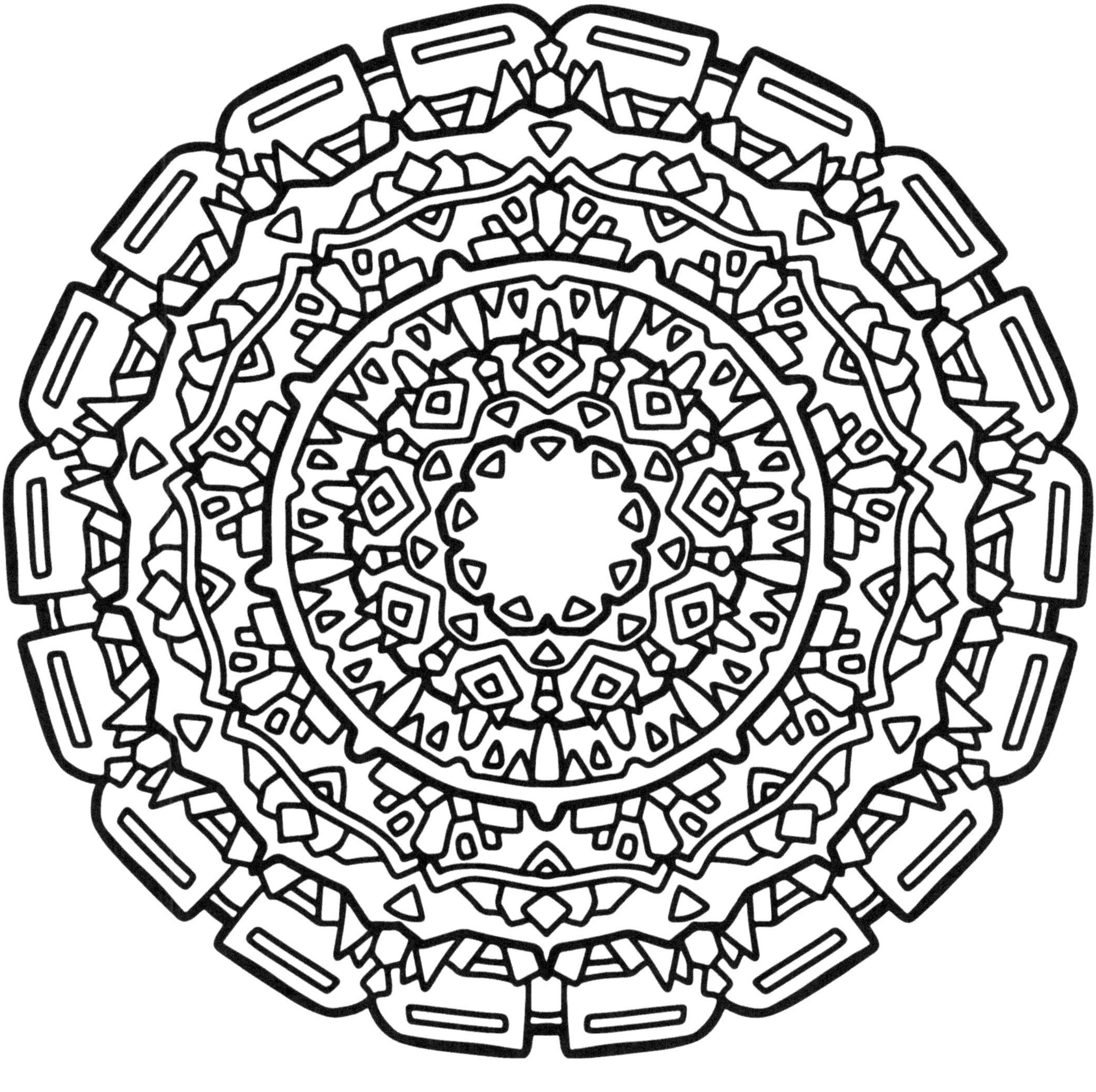

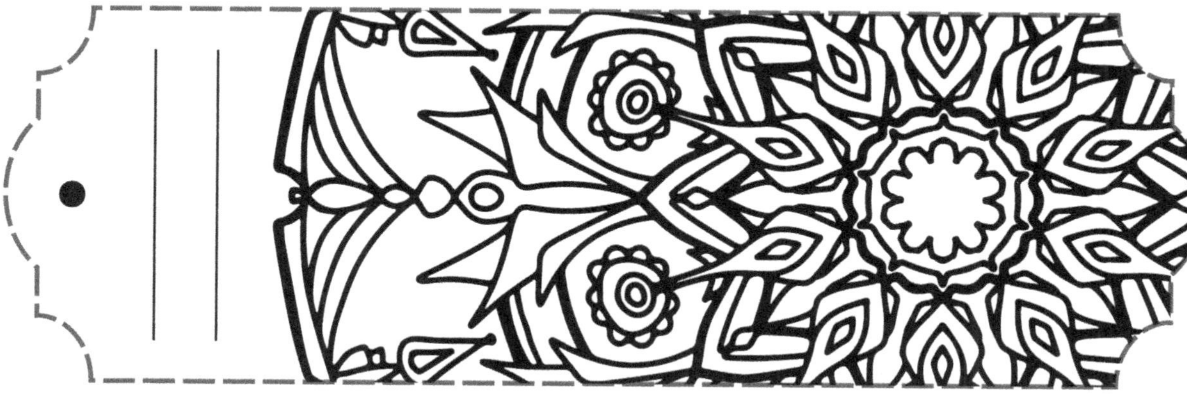

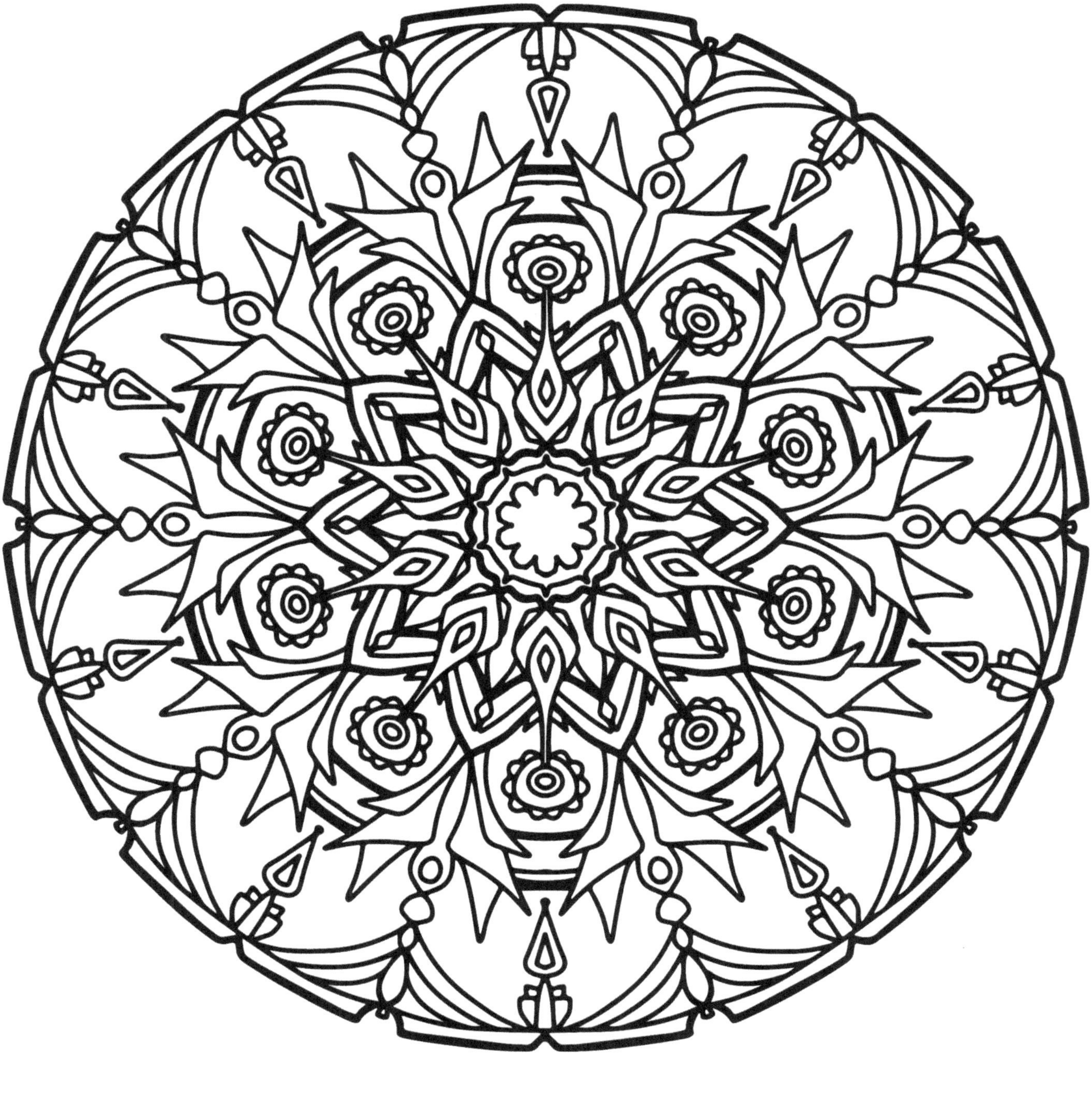

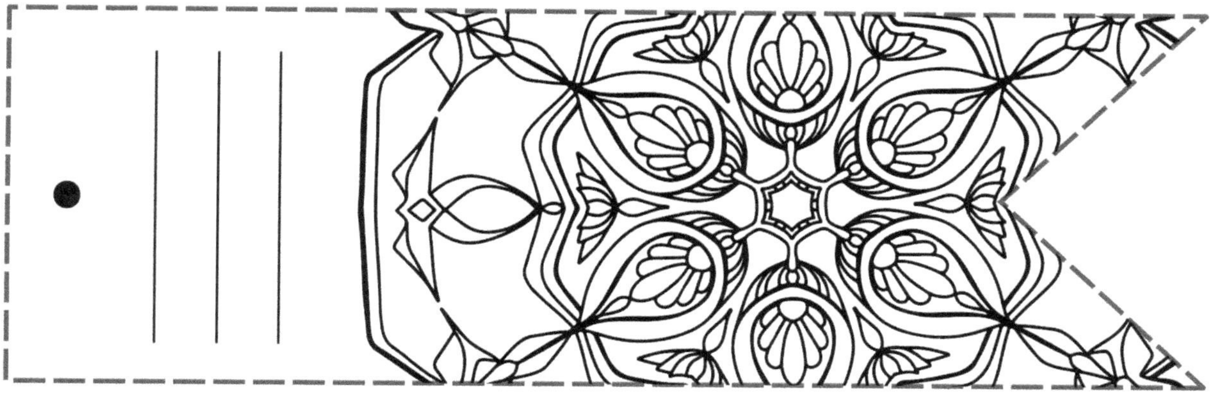

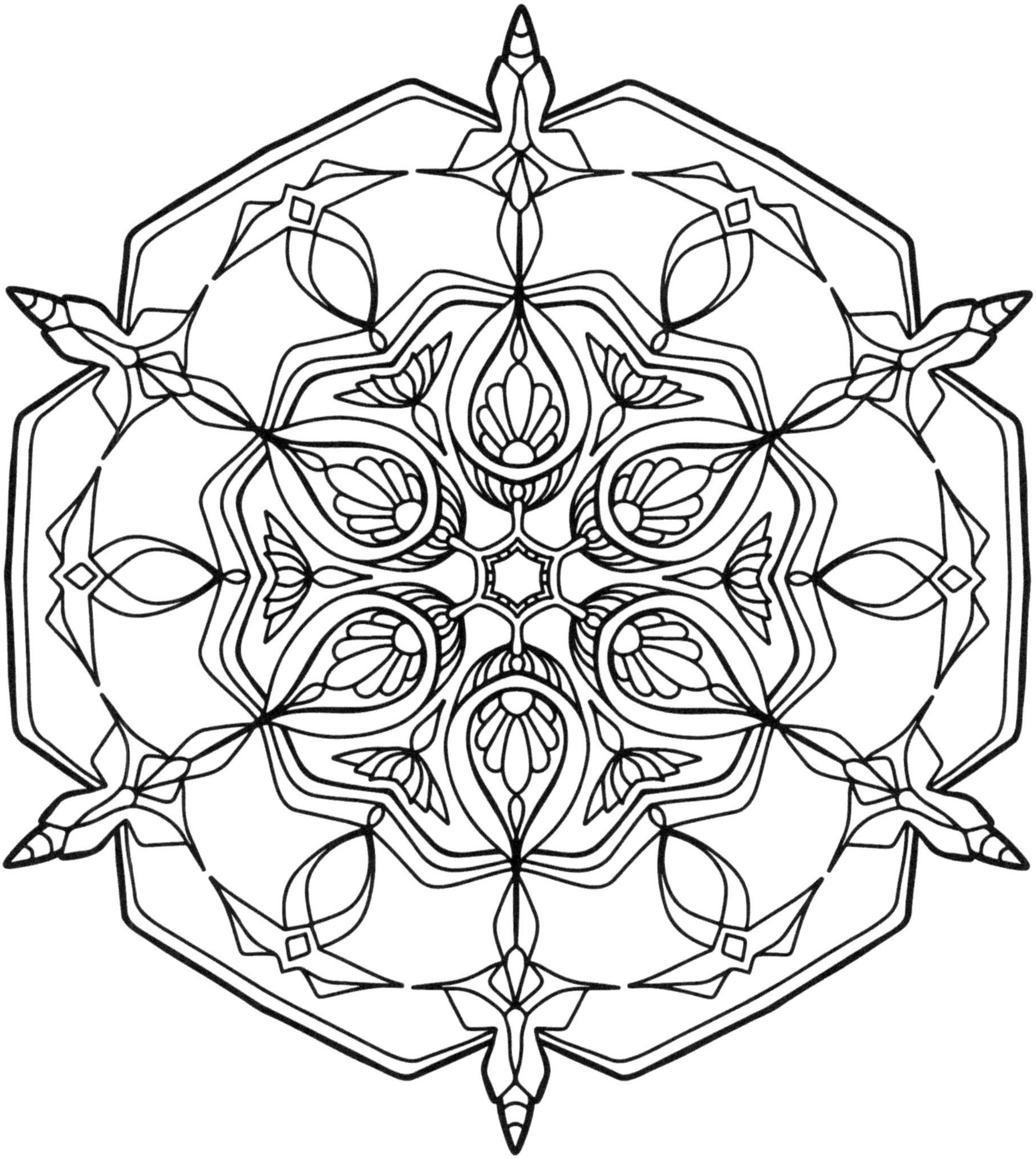

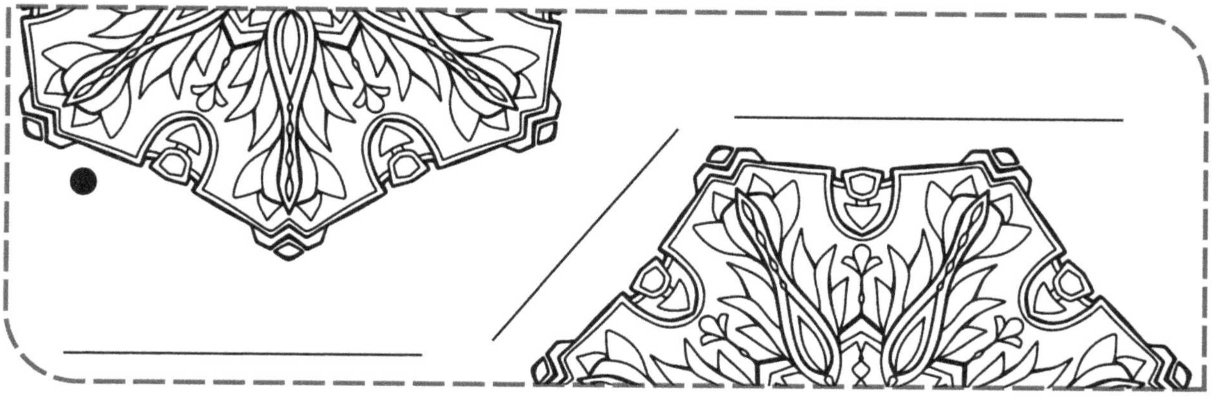

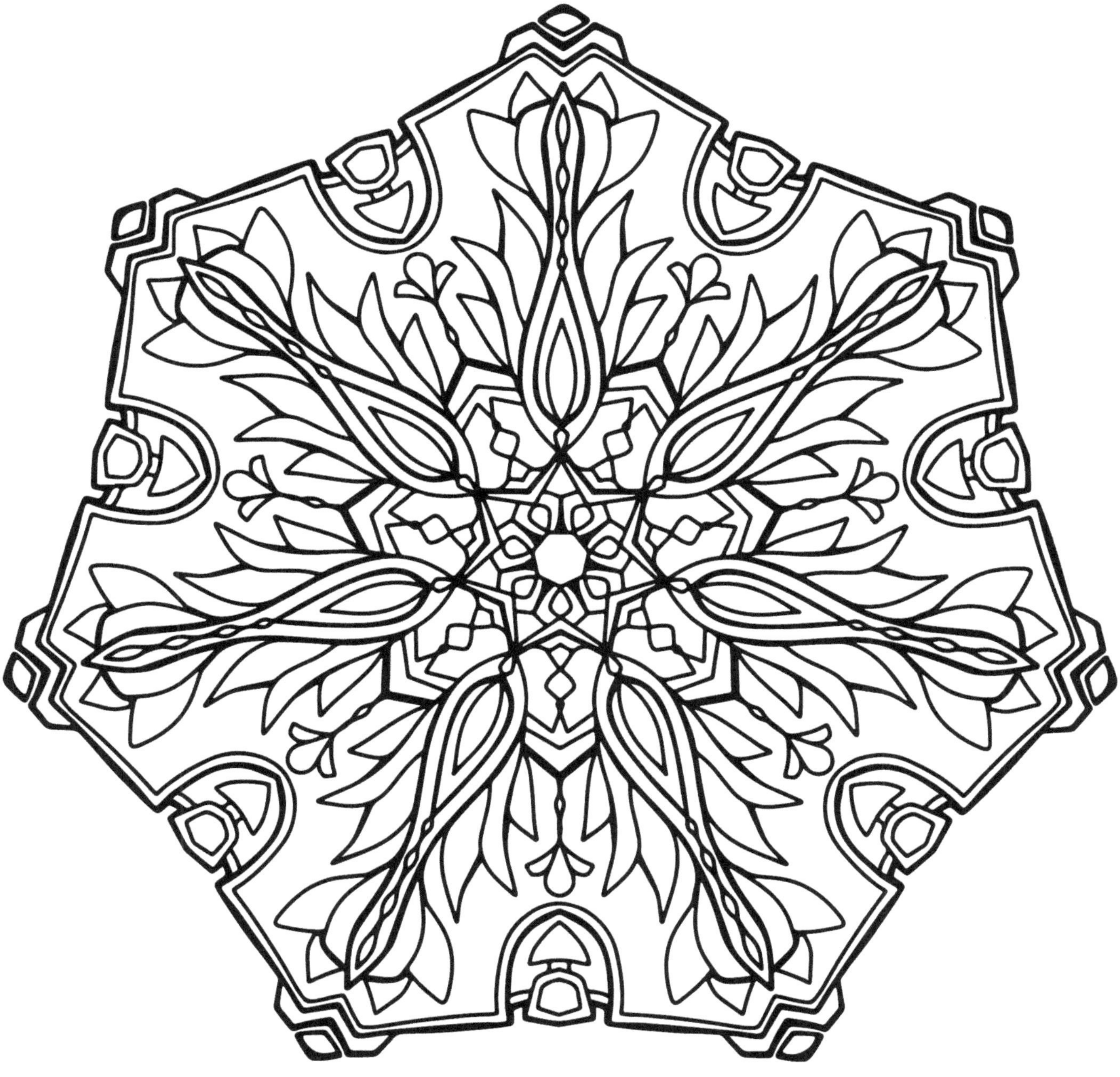

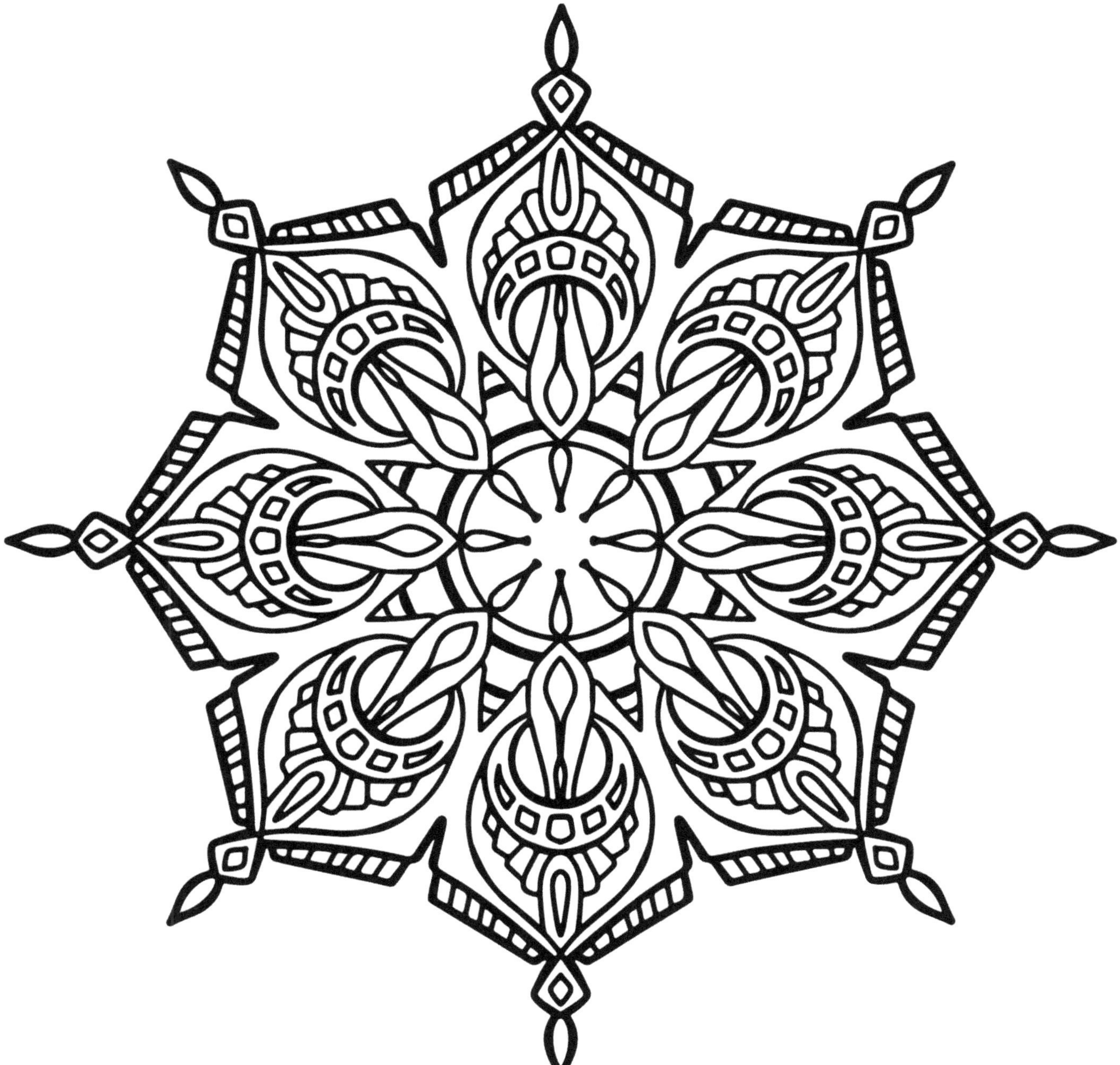

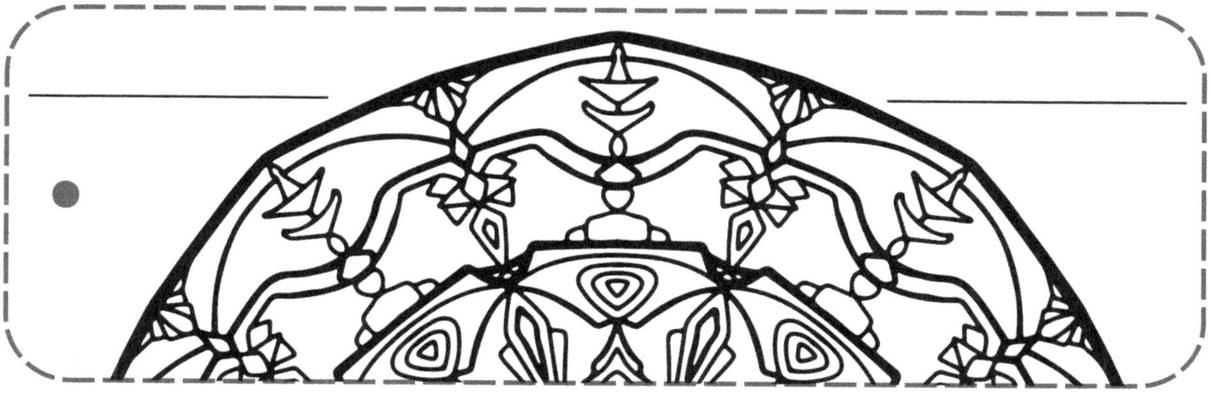

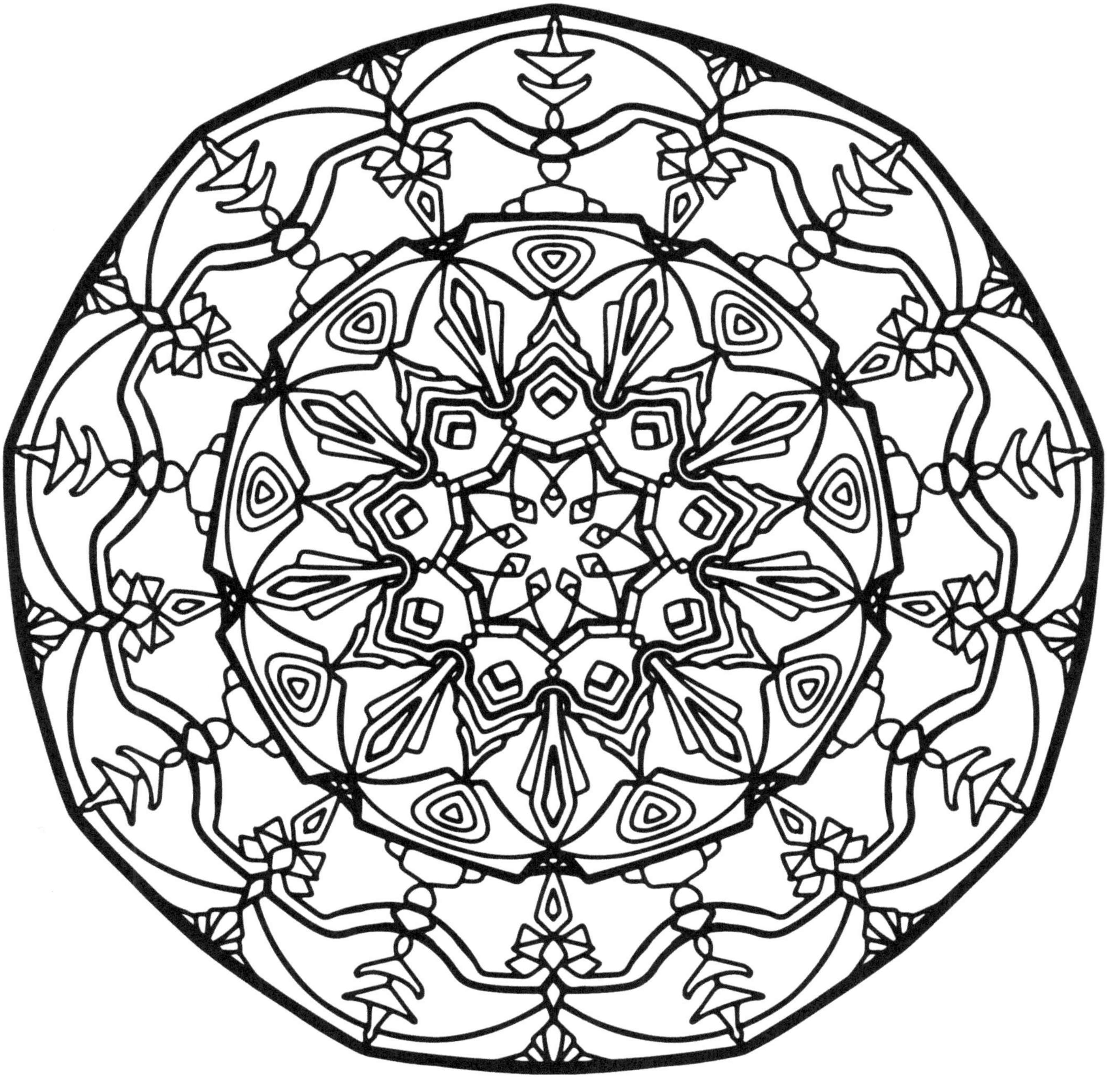

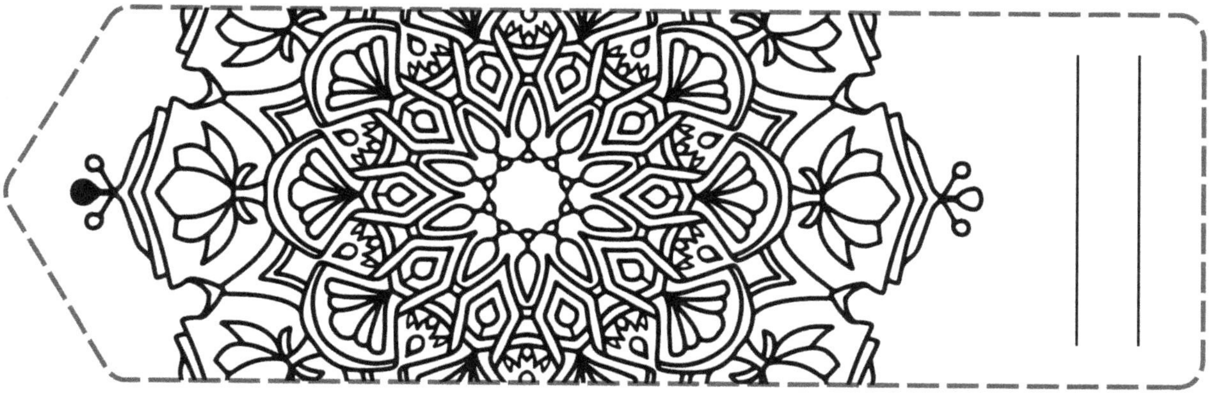

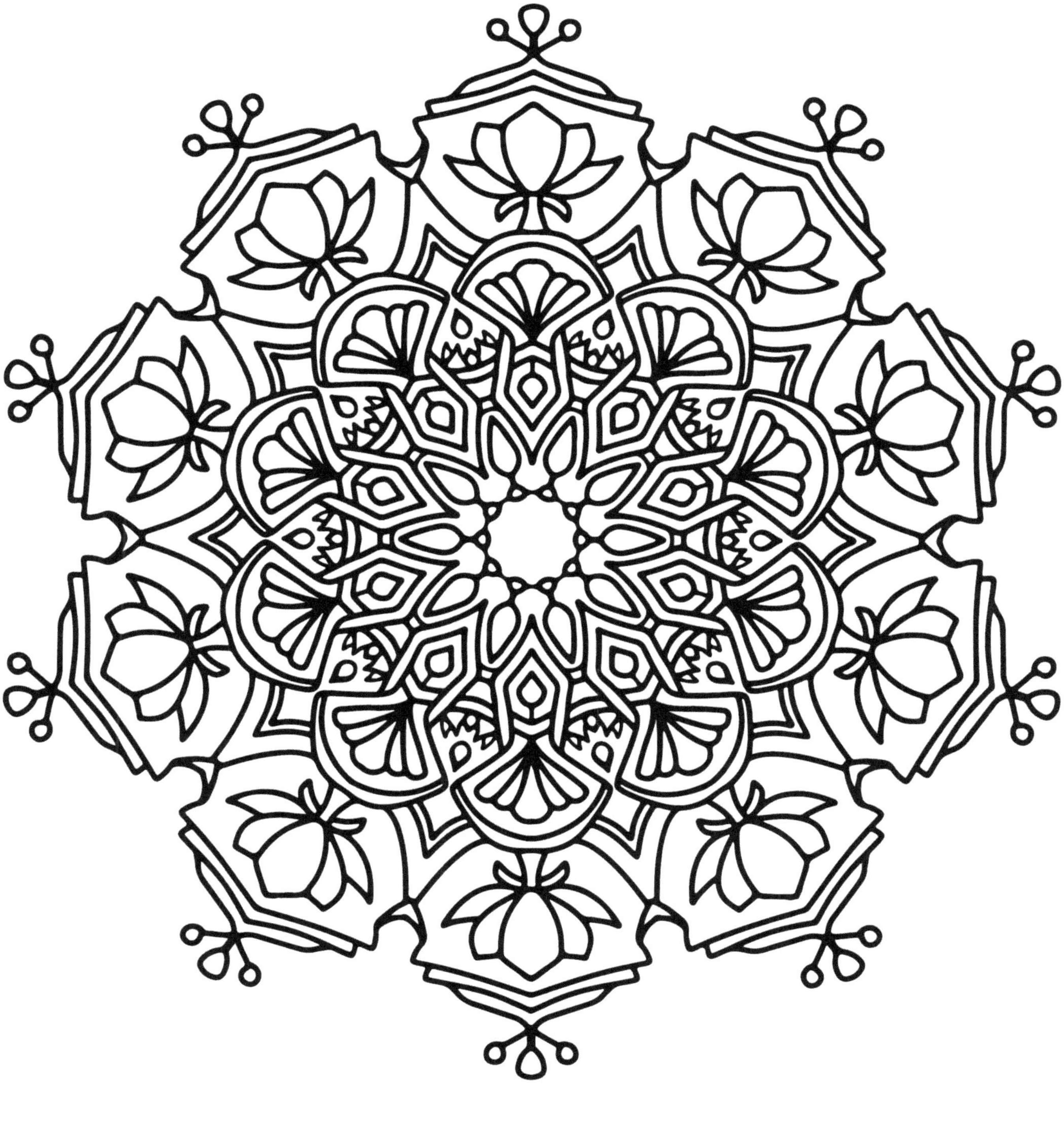

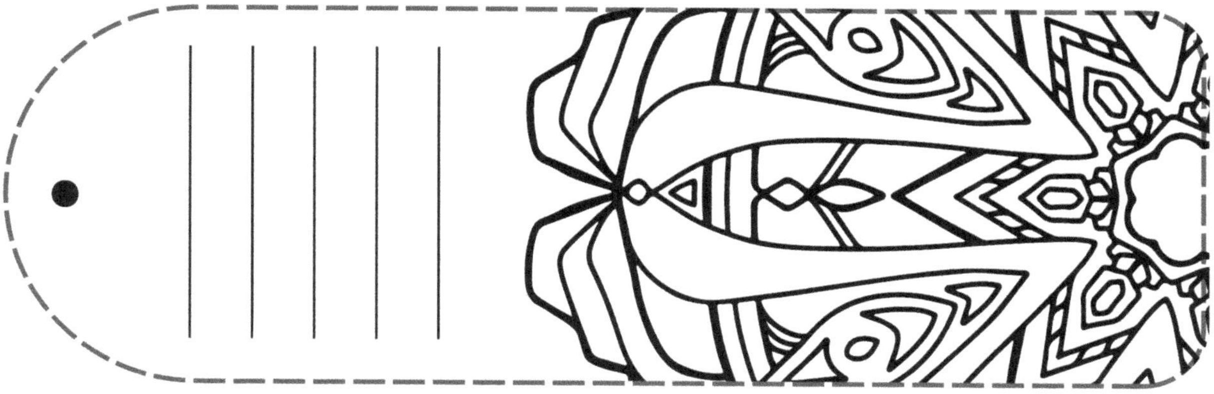

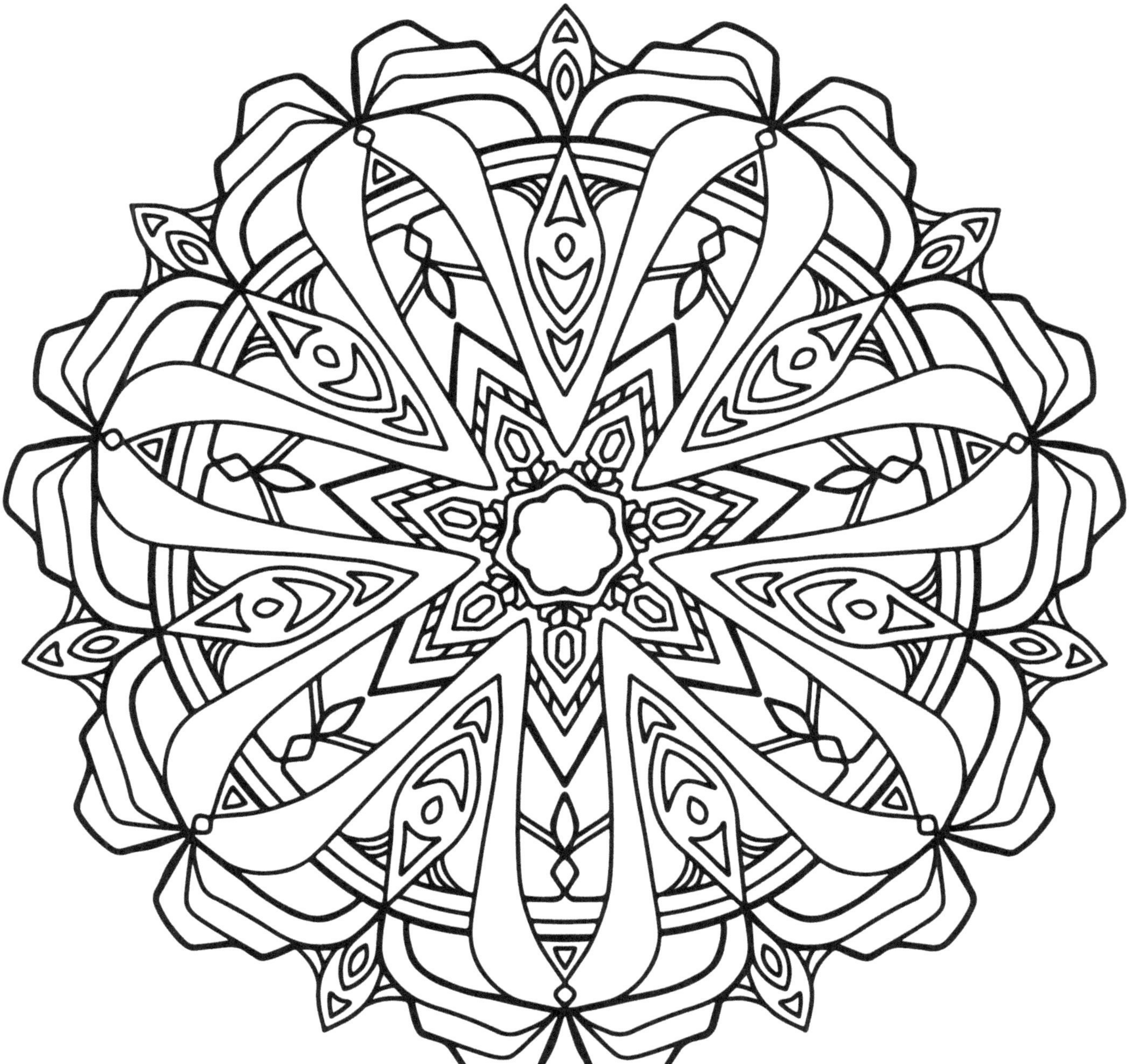

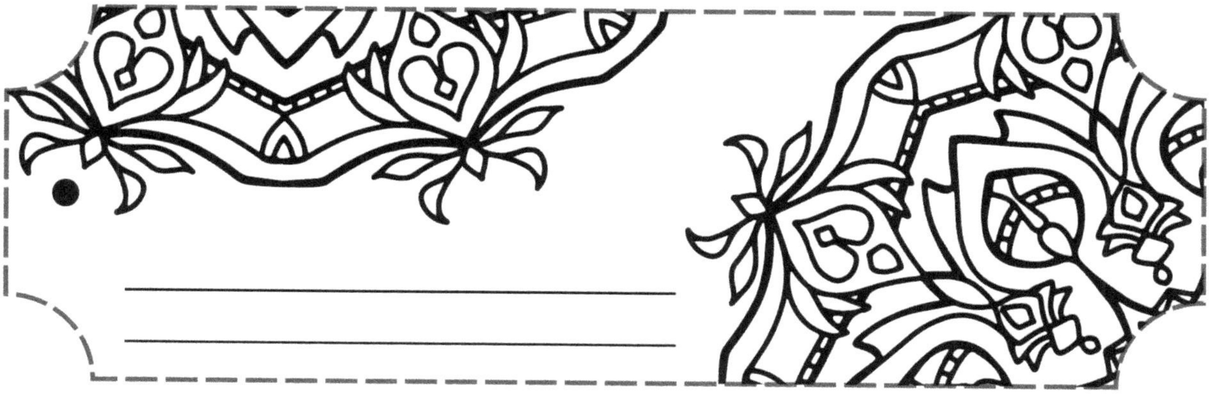

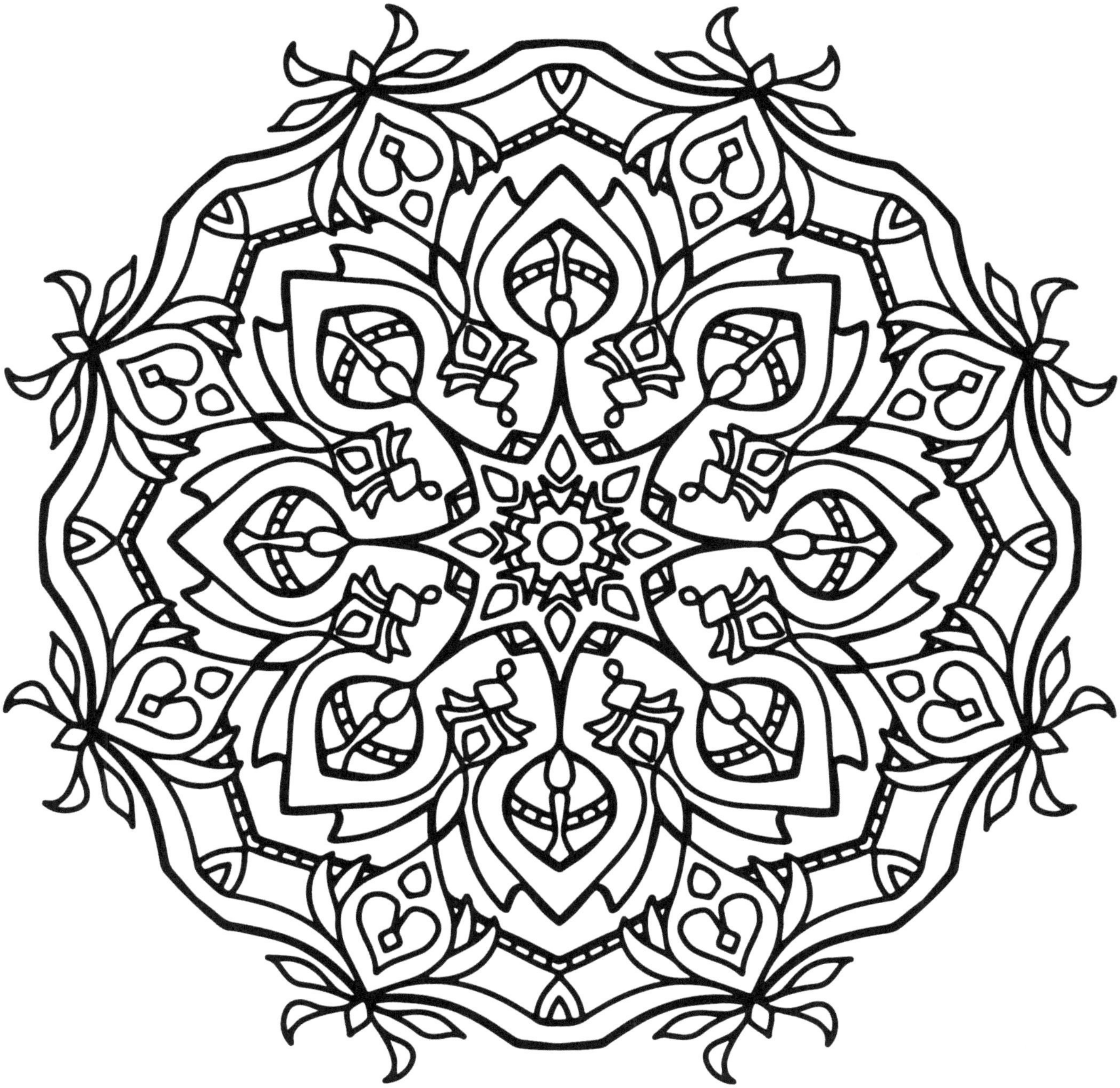

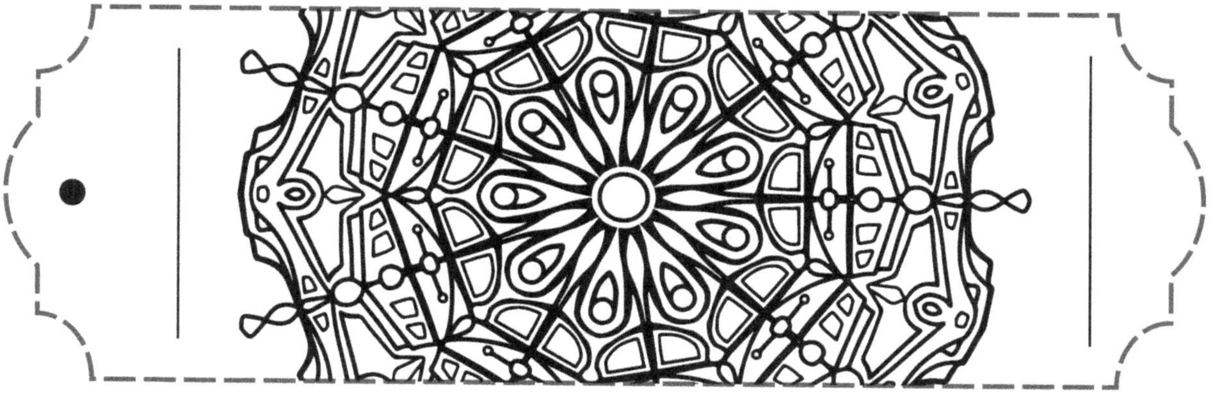

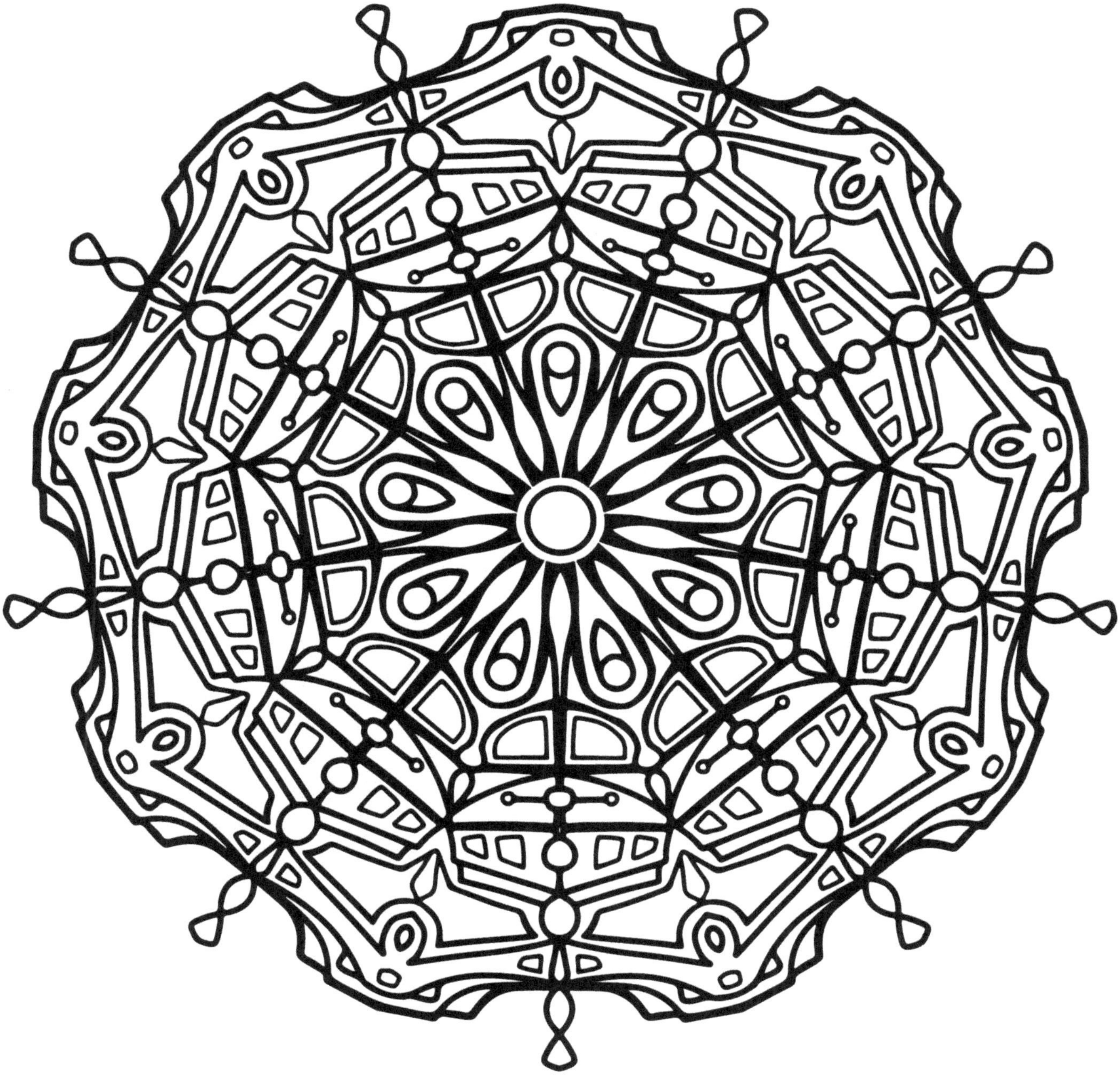

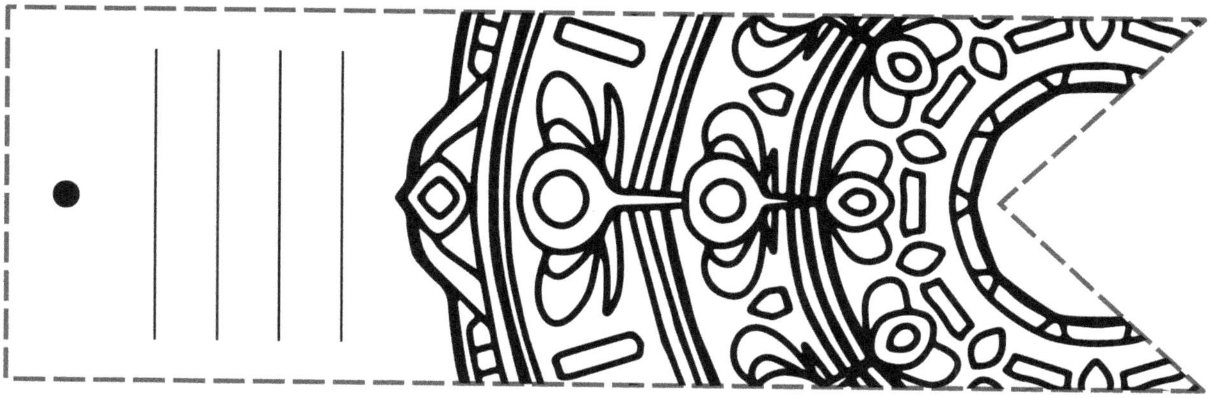

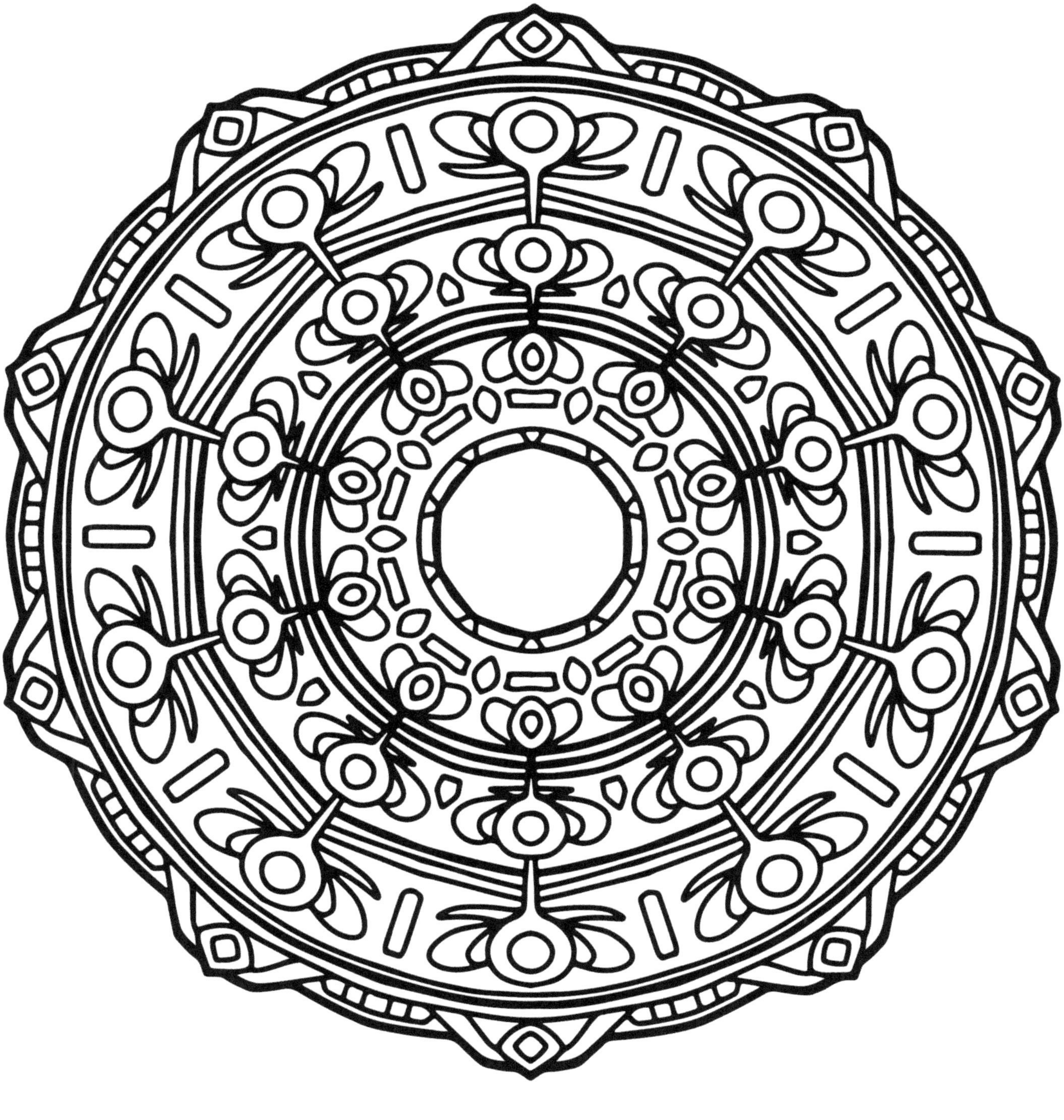

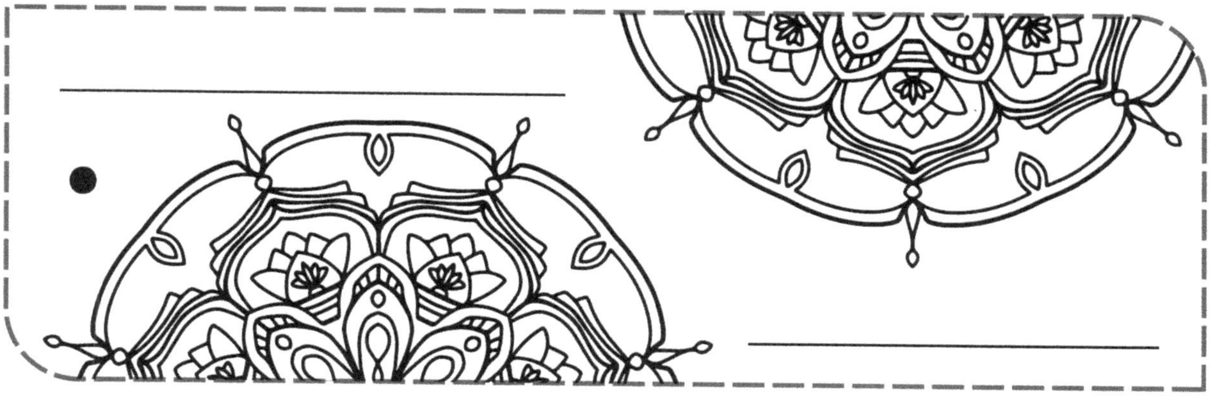

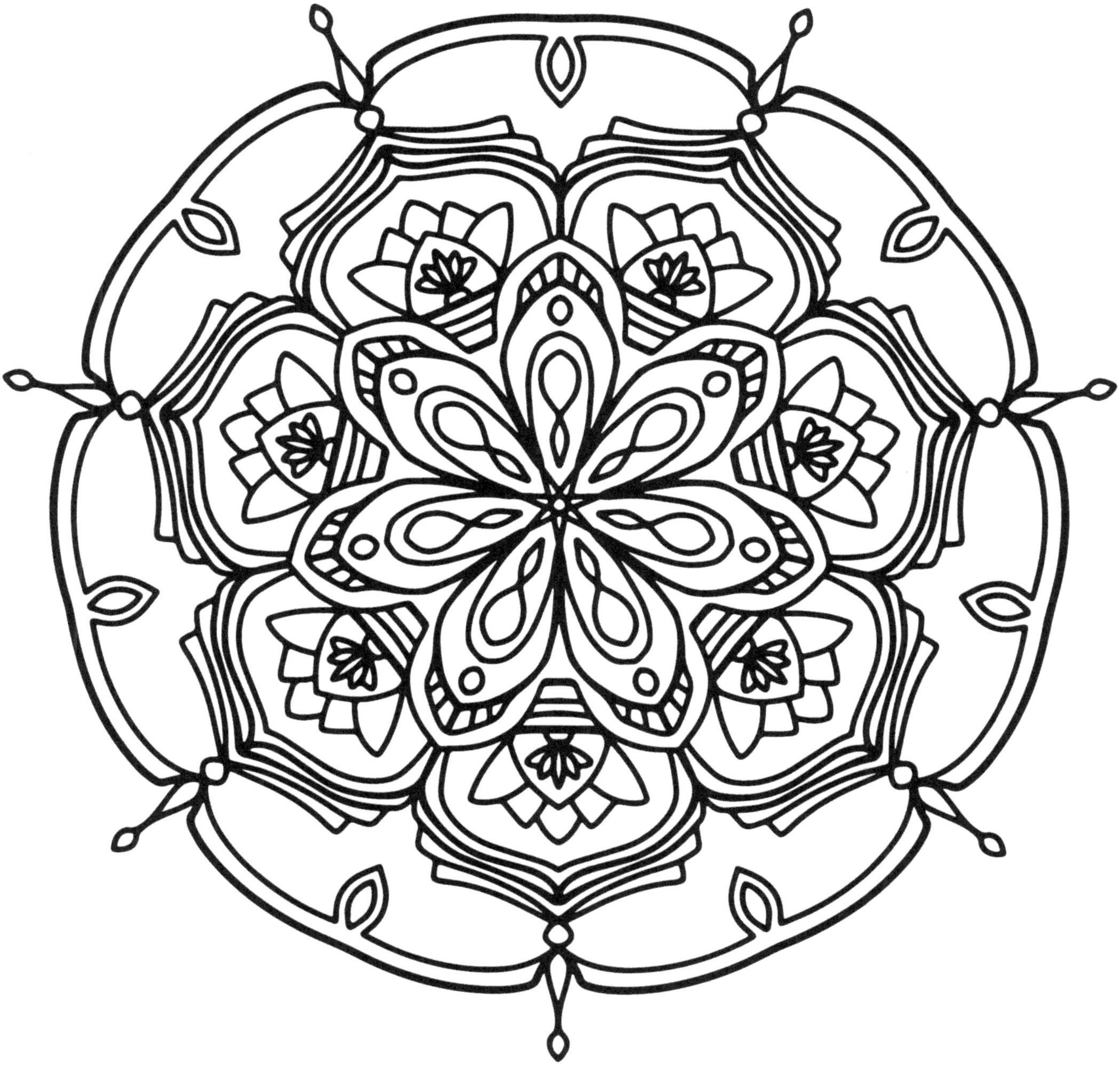

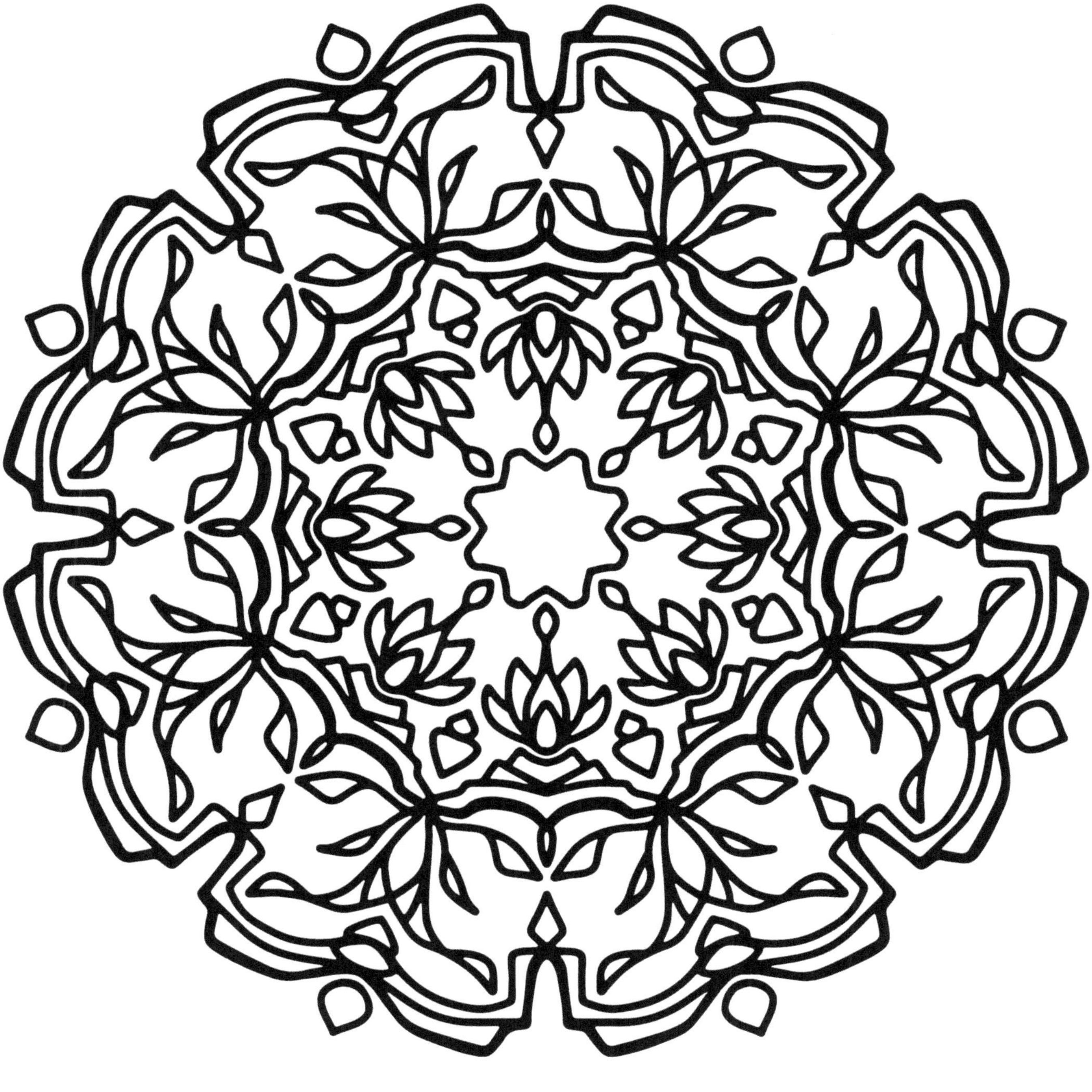

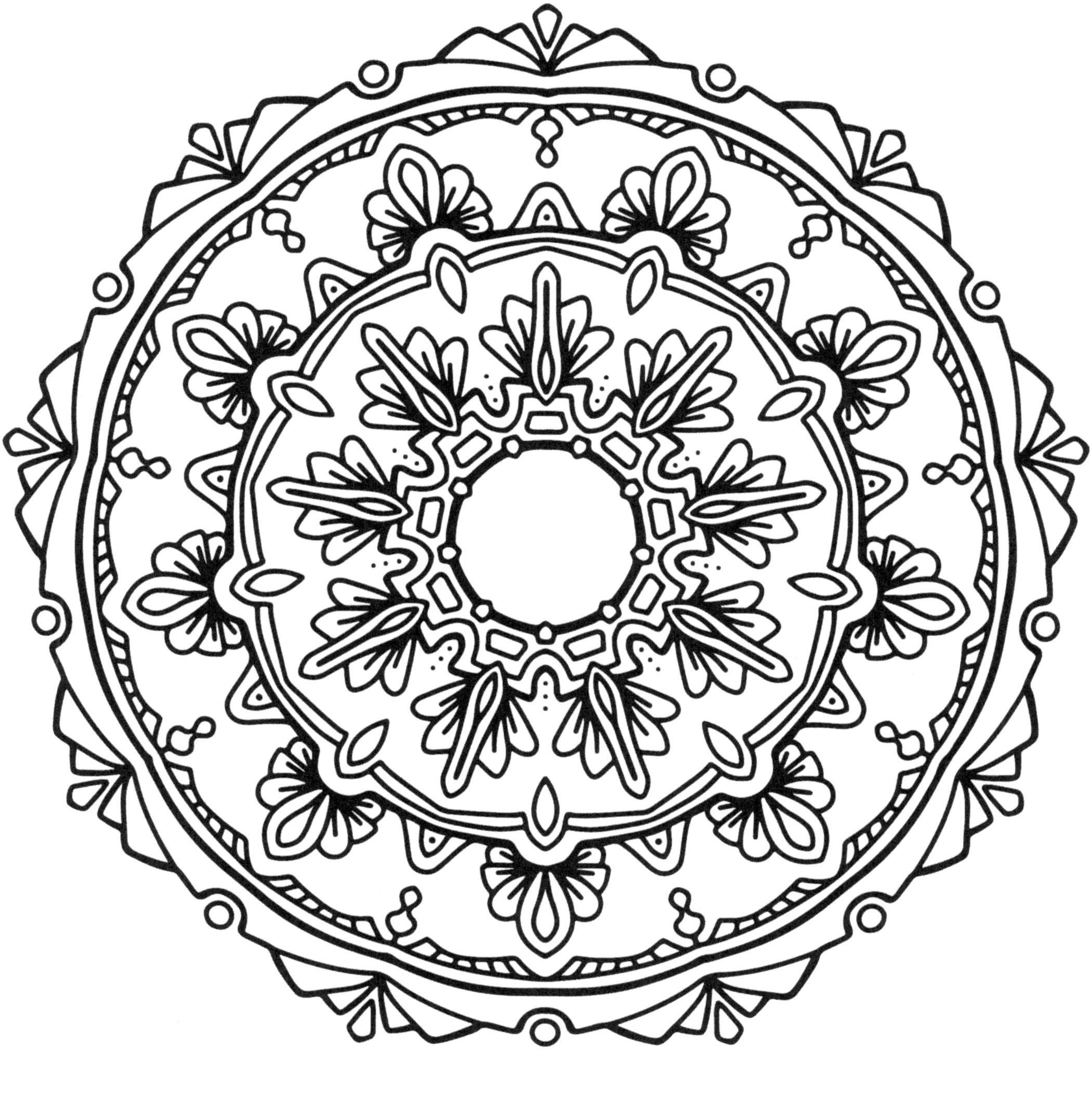

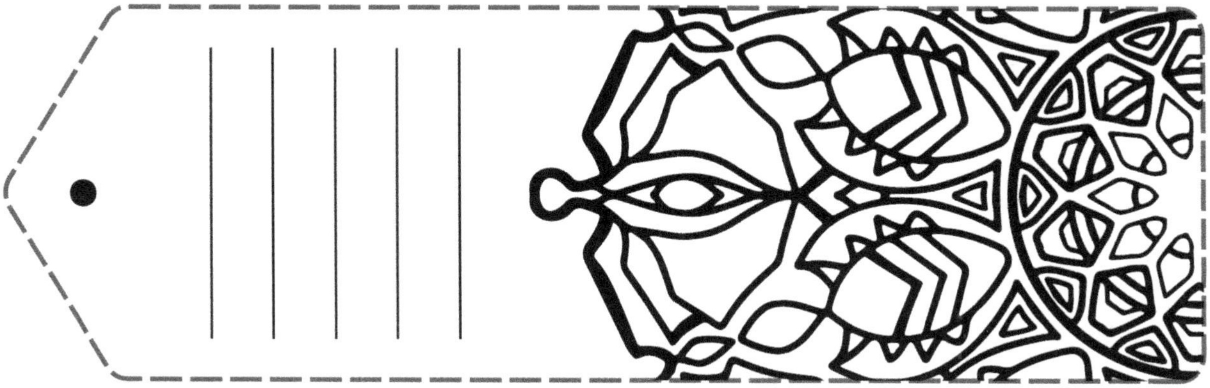

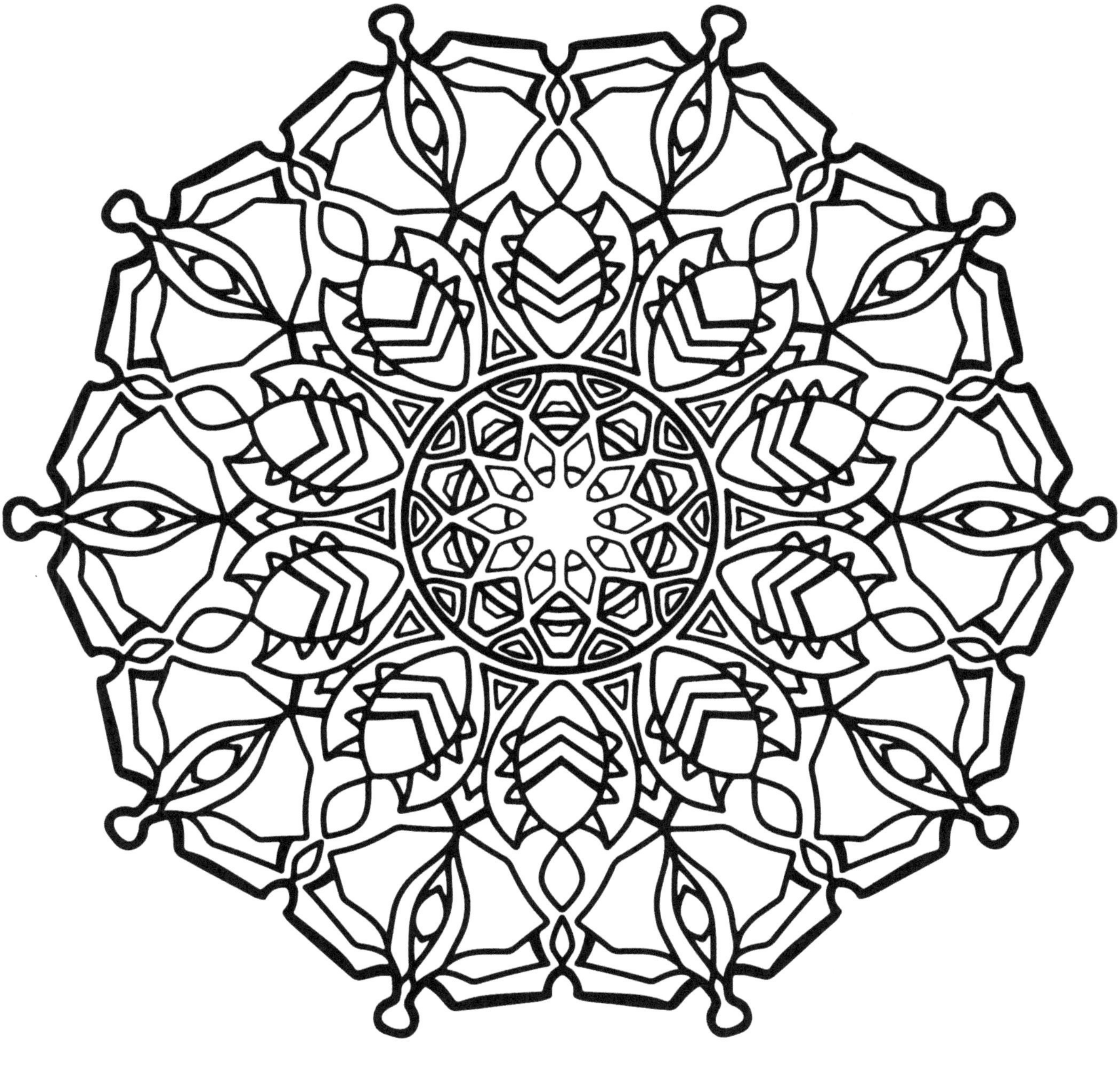

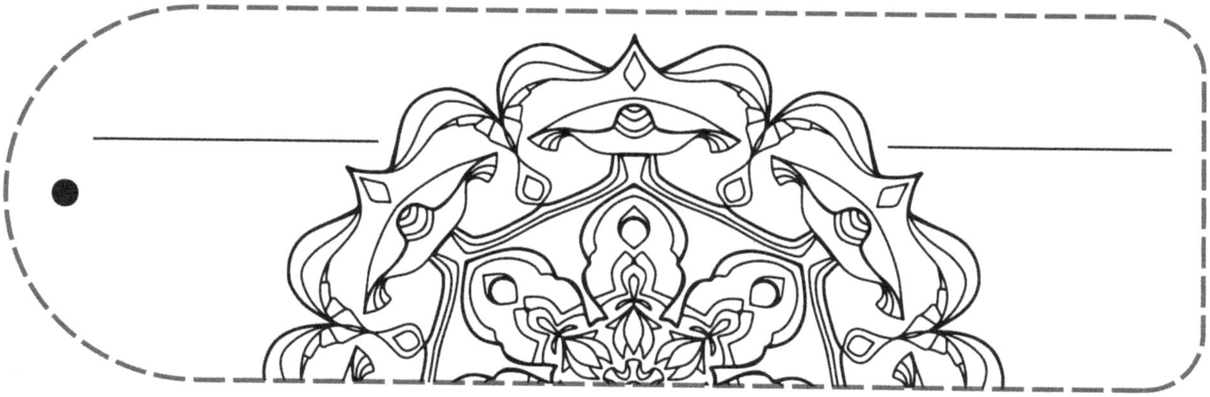

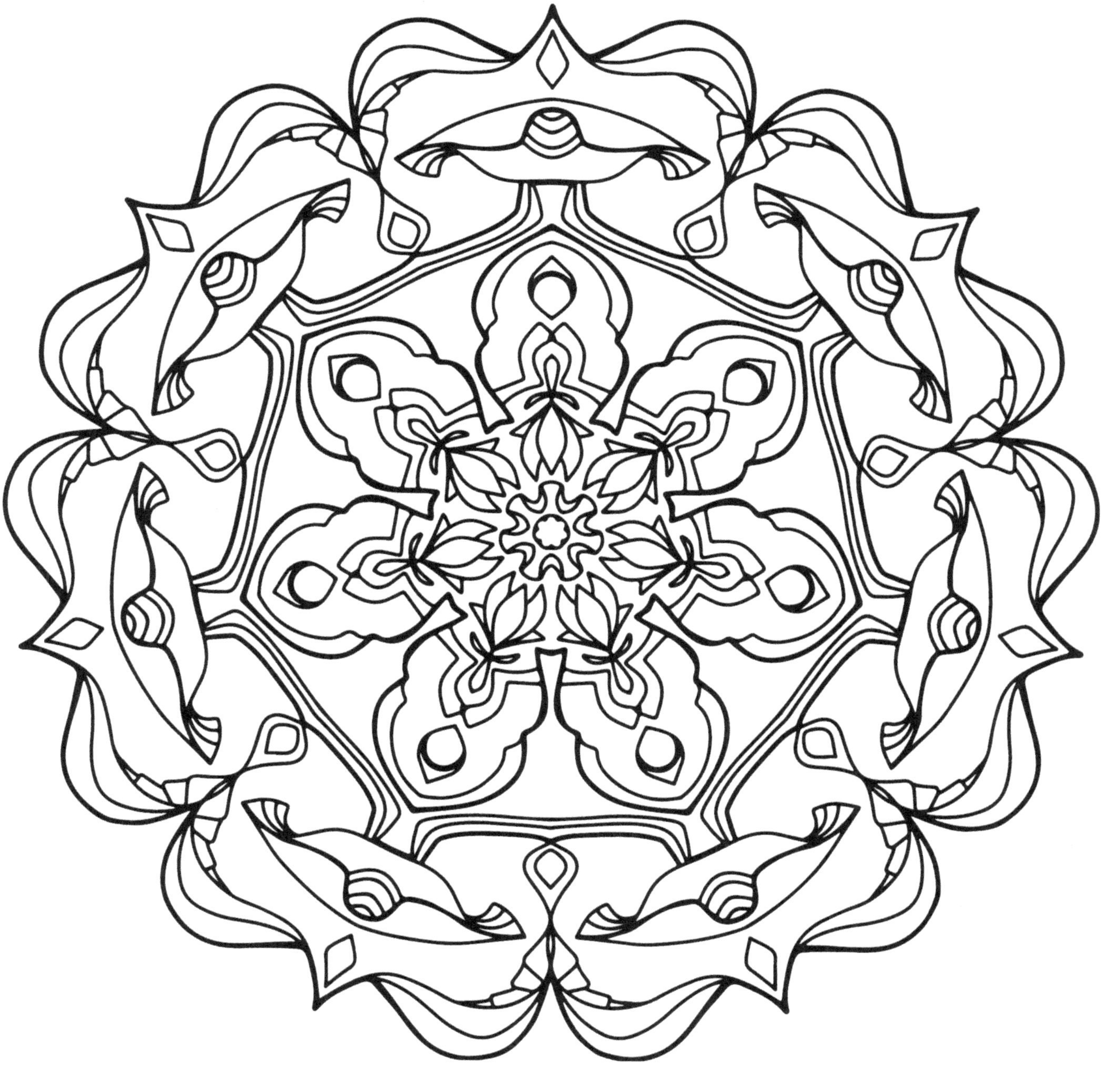

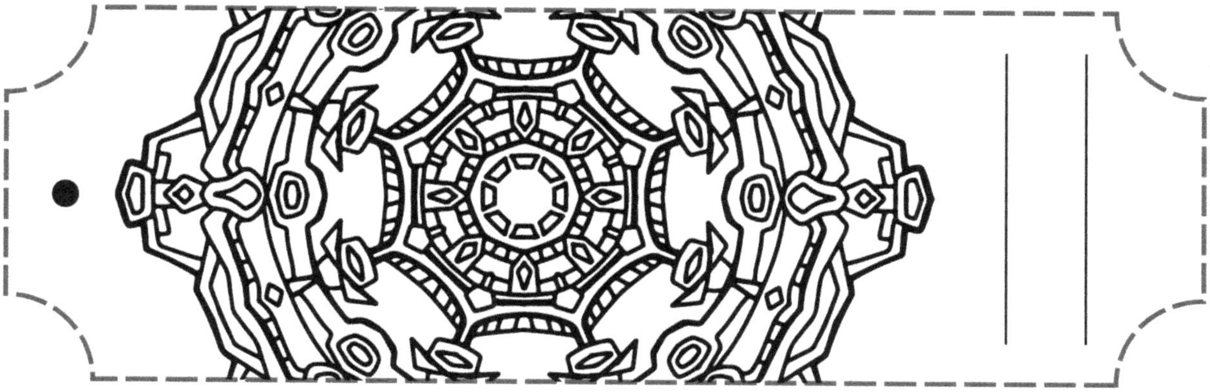

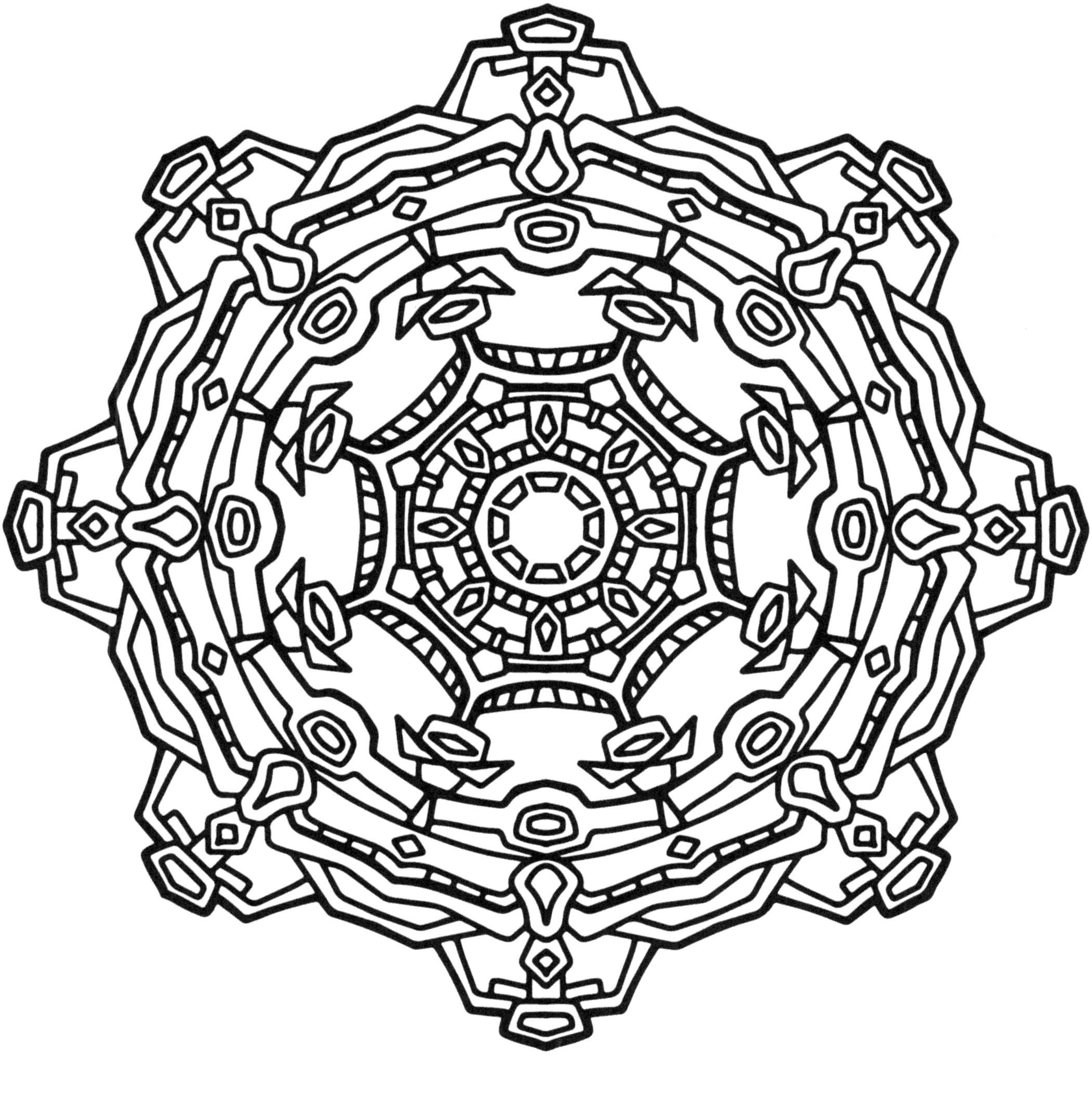

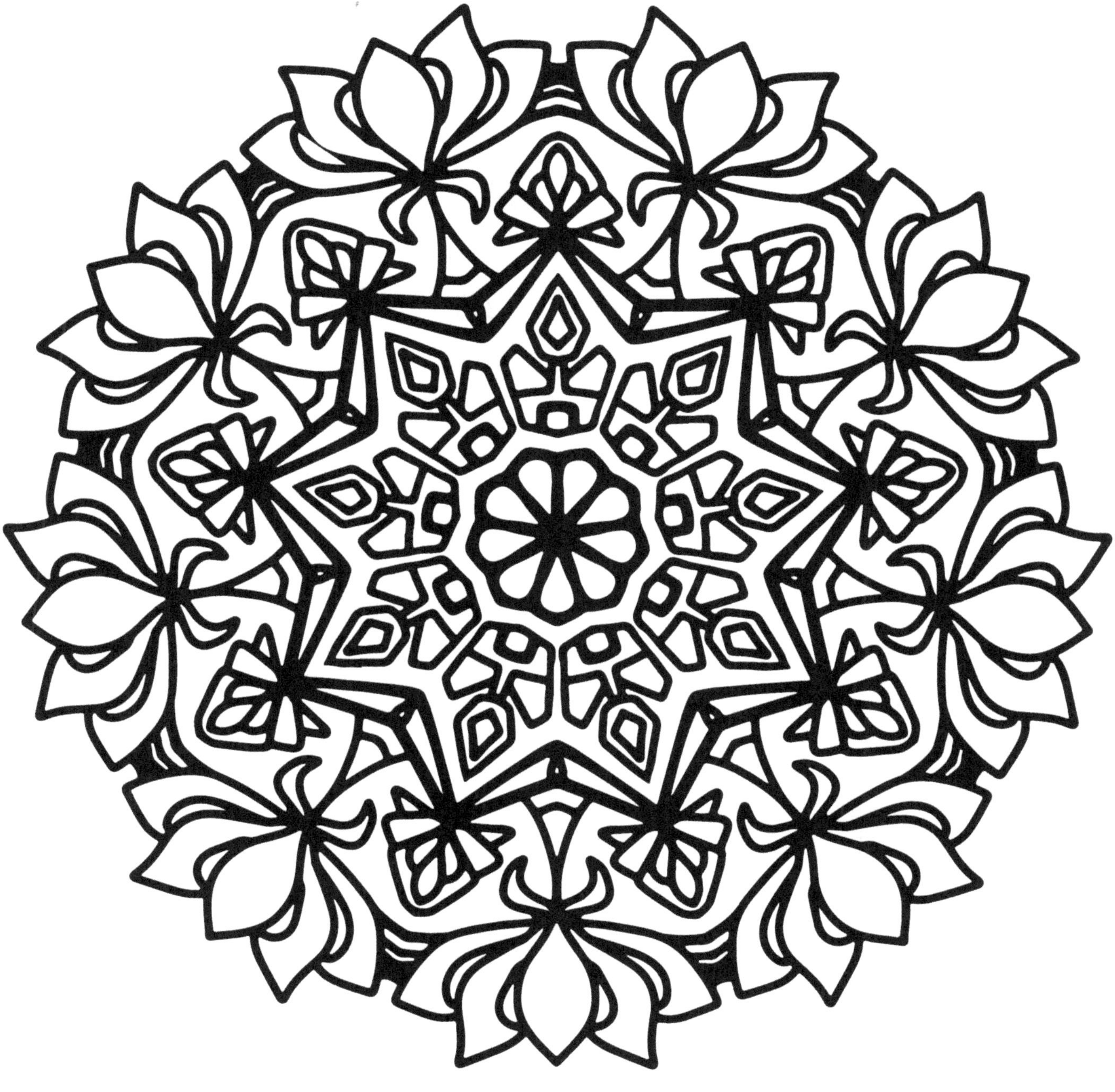

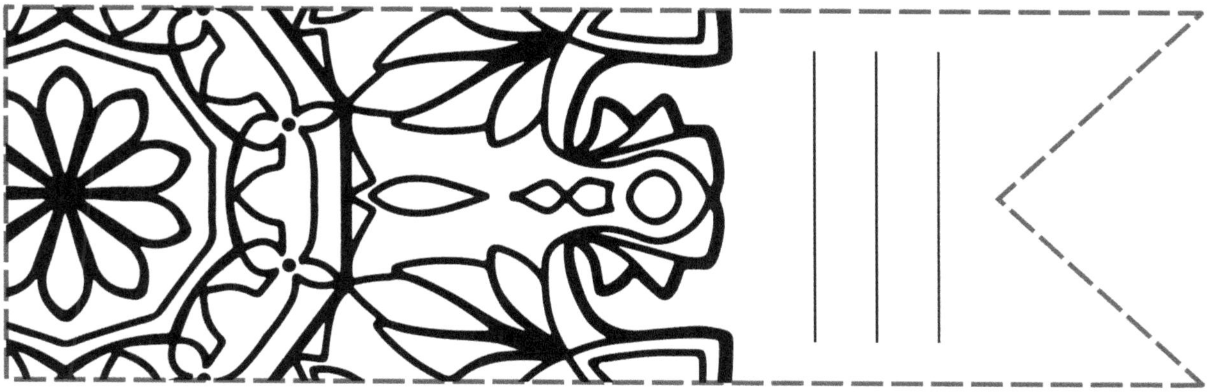

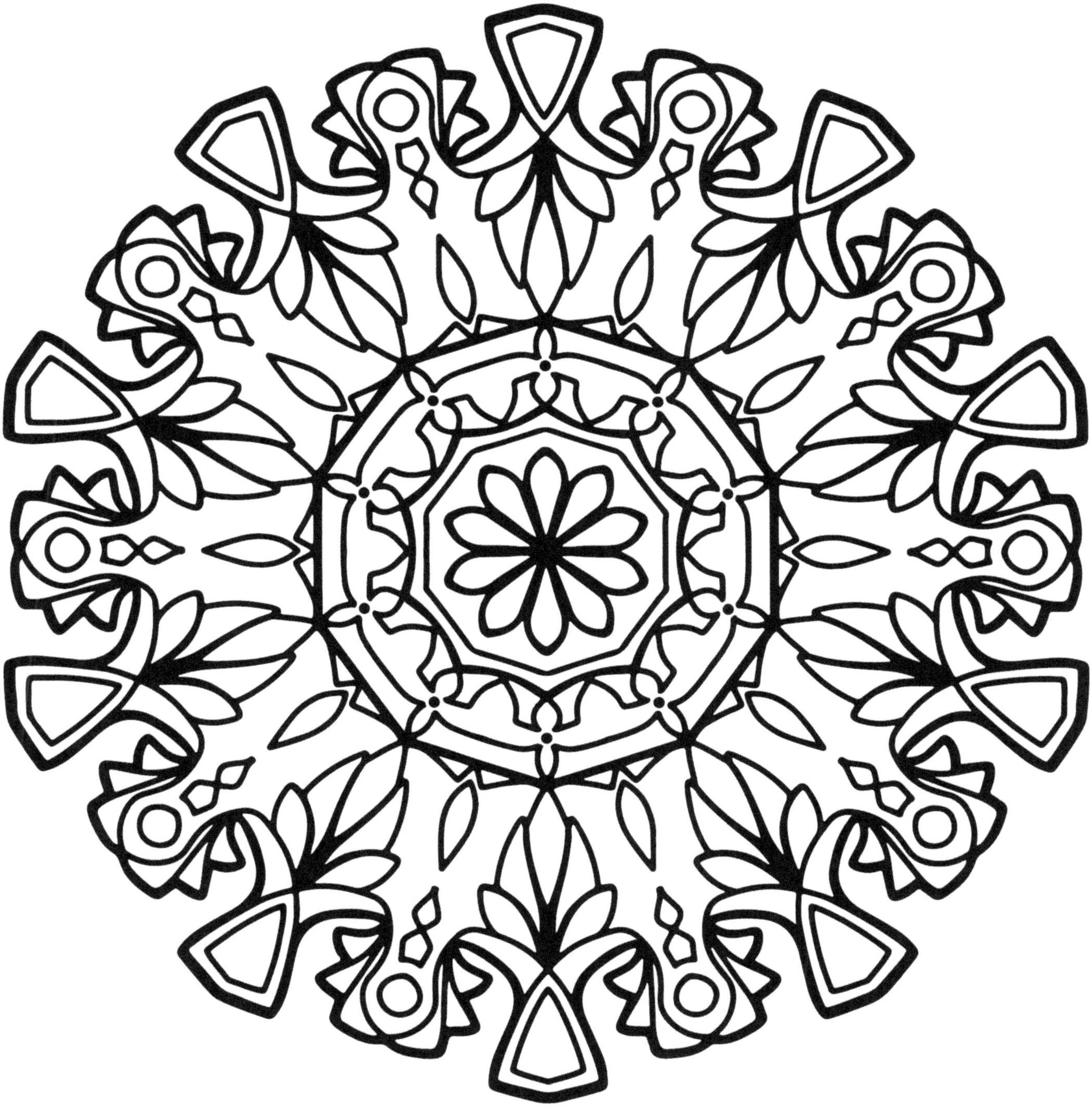

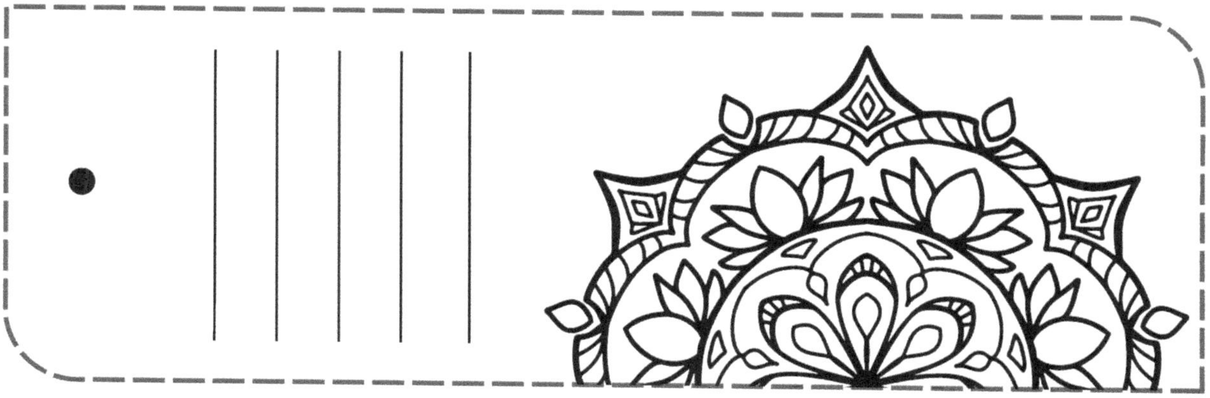

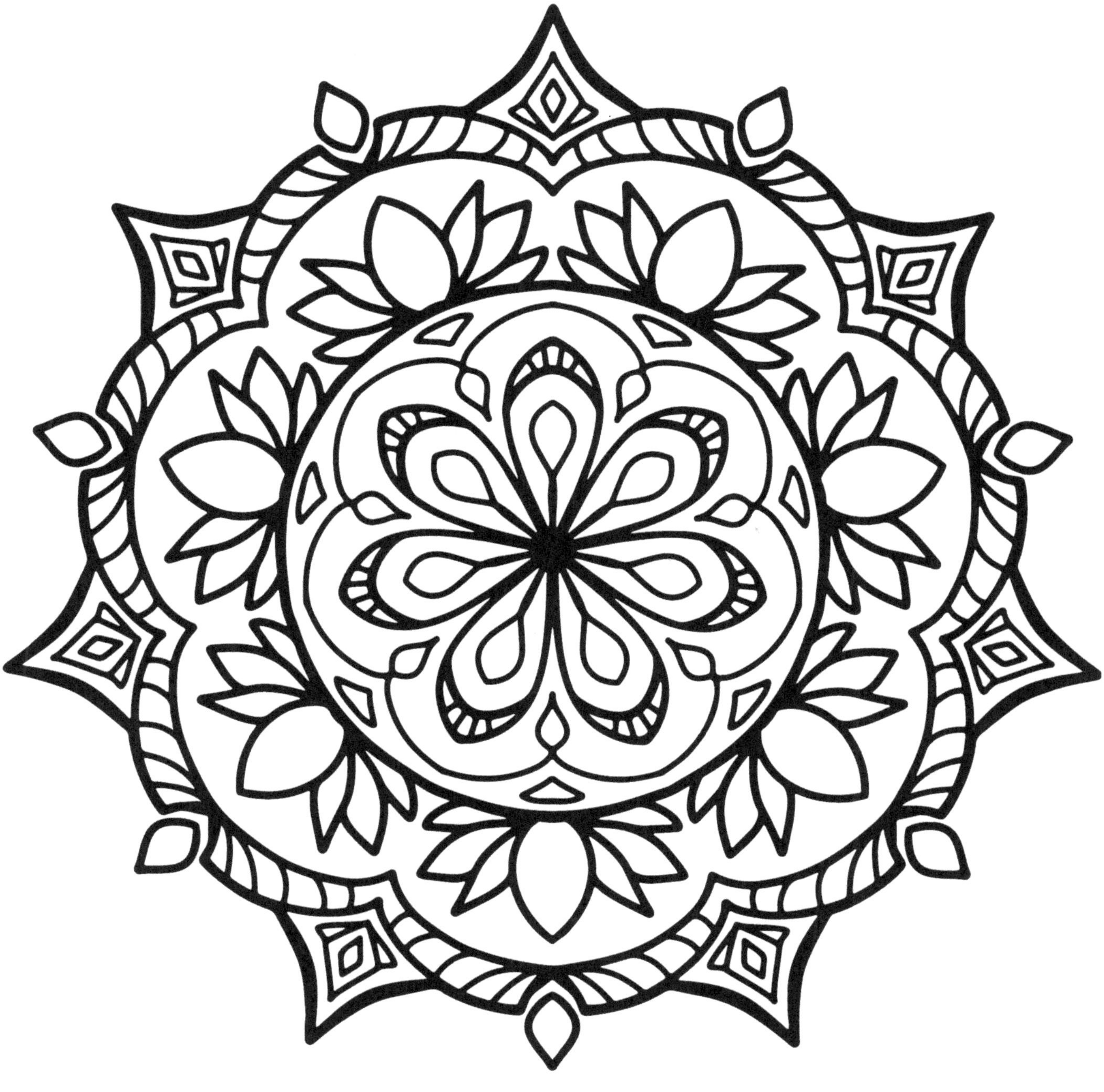

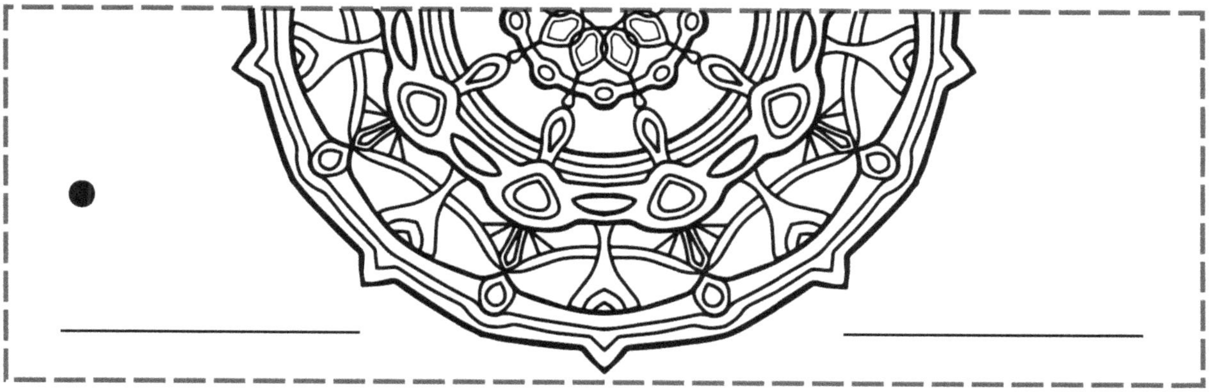

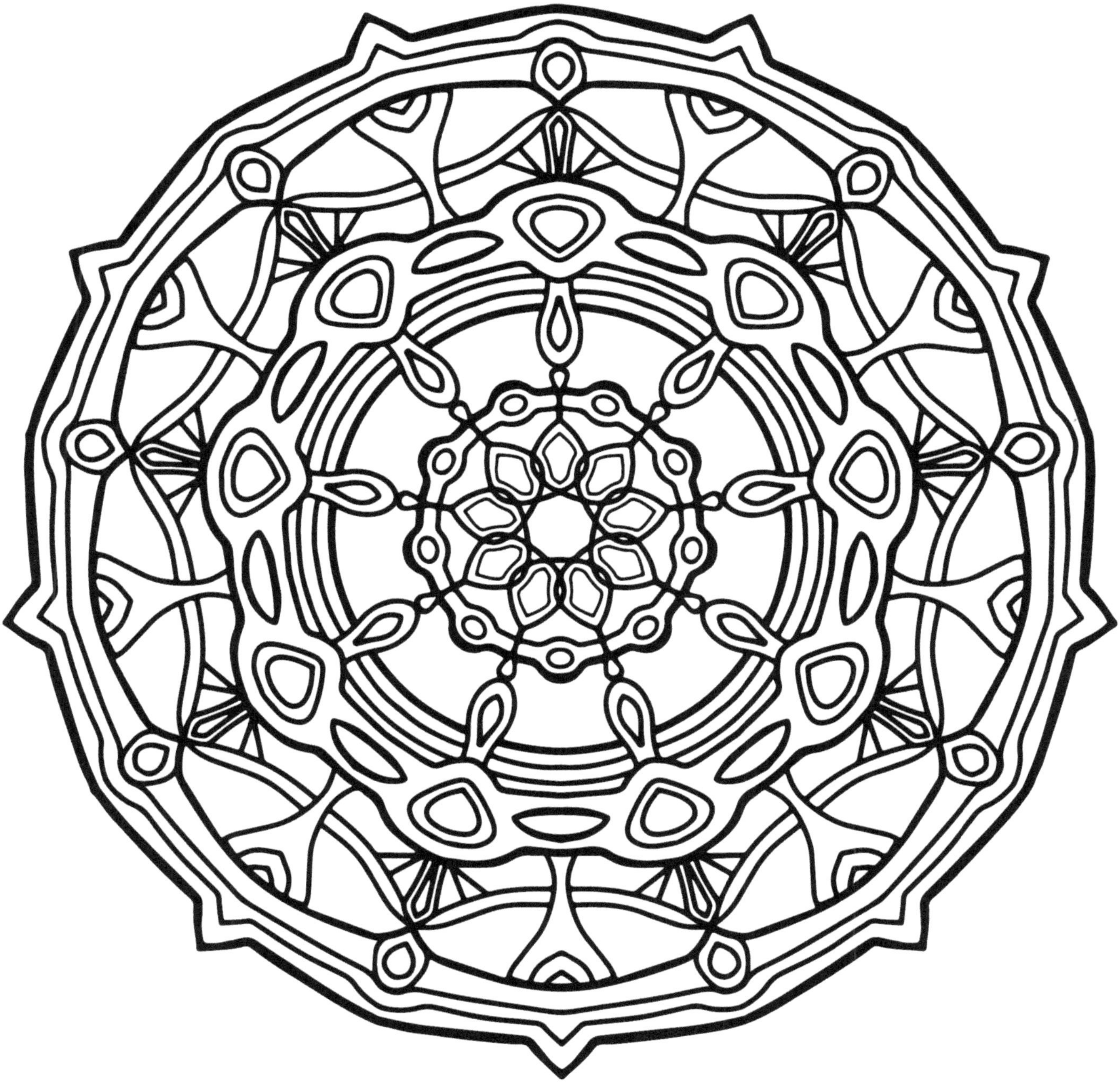

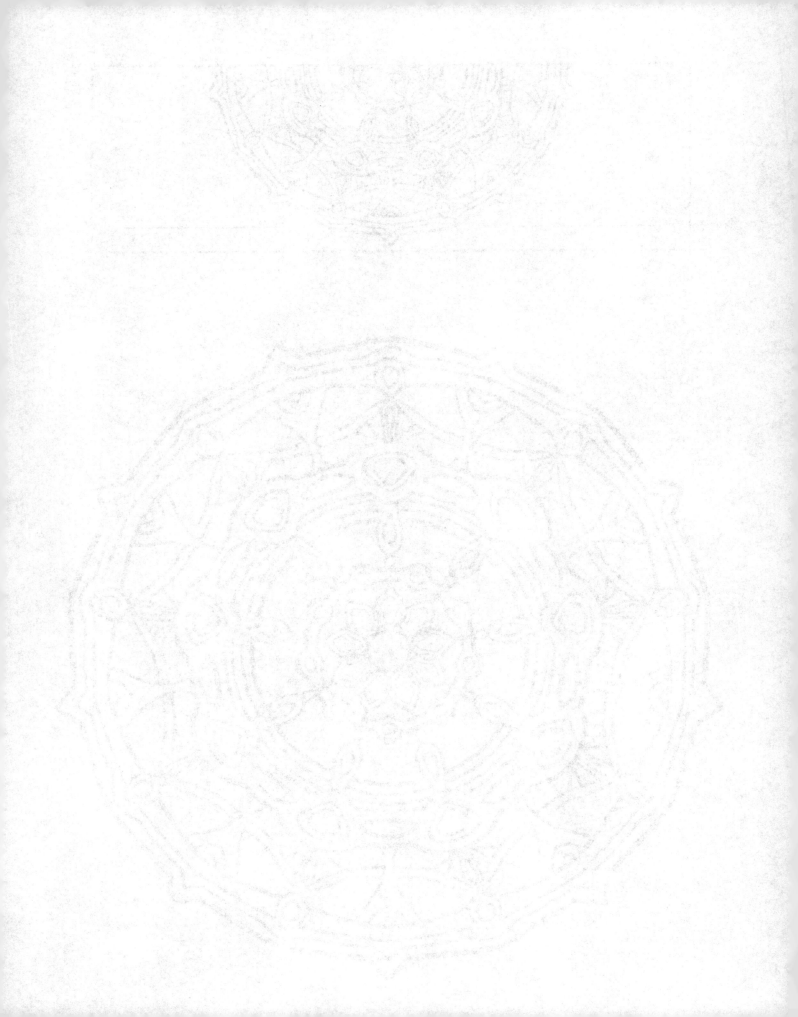

CPSIA information can be obtained
at www.ICGtesting.com
Printed in the USA
LVHW010349260121
677405LV00008B/191